new
pregnancy
and birth handbook

Dr.**miriam**
stoppard
MD FRCP

LONDON, NEW YORK, MUNICH
MELBOURNE, DELHI

For my sister, Hazel

Revised edition

Publishing Director Corinne Roberts
Brand Manager for Dr. Miriam Stoppard Lynne Brown
Senior Managing Editor Jemima Dunne
Project Editor Teresa Pritlove
Senior Art Editor Helen Spencer
Designer Ross George
DTP Designer Traci Salter
Production Kevin Ward

First published by Dorling Kindersley in 1985
This revised edition published in Great Britain in 2005 by Dorling
Kindersley Limited, 80 Strand, London WC2R ORL
A Penguin Company

A CIP catalogue record is available from the British Library.

ISBN 1-4053-0695-5

Contents

Introduction

It's a long time since I wrote my first book on pregnancy and childbirth and much has changed since then. One of the most important and welcome changes is the switch from doctor-supervised pregnancy and labour to one in which midwives play a major role. The concept of the "team" midwife is now adopted everywhere. Within this scheme of working, the antenatal and postnatal wards and the team of midwives on these combined wards remains the same. This ensures a continuity of care in which you'll be seen by the same group of midwives during your antenatal care, labour and postnatal recovery, making pregnancy and hospital birth happier and more relaxed than it has been in the past.

Fathers

THERE'S MUCH RESEARCH to show that if men are involved from the moment pregnancy's confirmed they become active and enthusiastic fathers. This means being involved in all the preparations, attendance at antenatal classes and clinics, in decisions as to where and how to have the baby, and with the care of the baby from day one. If men are shut out at any stage, the role of father is more difficult to assimilate. There's no greater help to a pregnant woman than an interested and sympathetic partner. There's no better medical attendant in the delivery room than an understanding, supportive father and there's certainly no better help with a newborn baby than an active, passionate dad. The labour itself can be just as remarkable an experience for the father as it is for the mothers.

A major priority for a pregnant woman is to have adequate help and while the best help may be a partner, it doesn't have to be. It may be more practical and even more emotionally supportive to have a close friend or relation – your mother or sister for instance – to be your birth assistant. An option you might like to exercise is having both your partner and a friend with you during labour. To clear this path necessitates long-term planning and involvement from the beginning for all concerned with your antenatal classes, your visits to hospital, and chats to midwives and nursing staff about how your labour will be conducted. As you can imagine this isn't always straightforward, but the book will help you to pick your way through various possibilities.

Approaching motherhood

FOR MANY WOMEN TODAY motherhood comes rather later in life than it used to. It's now commonplace for a woman to pursue her career into her thirties and decide to have her first child somewhere around 35. The old obstetric concept of being an "elderly primipara" after the age of 30 is now outdated. With improvements to overall maternal health, doctors and midwives are used to dealing with first-time mothers in their late thirties and even early forties as a matter of routine, and see these pregnancies as normal, rather than a cause for alarm.

Most women work for most of their pregnancy. Planning for a modern pregnancy and the birth is quite different from that in the past. Now most women feel they have to give careful consideration to their future job security and I've outlined the advantages and disadvantages in this book of combining work, pregnancy and motherhood. Even if you have planned to resume your job after say six months, you may find it impossible to leave your baby and decide to wait a few months longer. No one knows before the birth of their own child just how they will feel in the event.

Every woman is beset by doubts, fears and anxieties – you wouldn't be normal if you didn't have them. Yet it will all seem easy and straightforward in retrospect. In the meanwhile, it's reassuring to think about the women all around you, hardly different from yourself, who are enjoying pregnancies, having memorable labours and births and, despite some sleepless nights, worries about feeds and weight gain, are thrilled with their babies. You, like them, will find that pregnancy and birth introduce you to a fulfilling phase of your life.

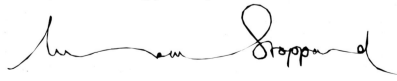

Pregnancy calendar

Knowing about the changes that happen during pregnancy helps you to become more aware of your body and your needs. It also helps you to remain calm if you understand that these changes, which aren't inevitable in all women, are perfectly normal. This month-by-month calendar summarizes the development of the baby and the changes in your body. However, every pregnancy is different; no two pregnancies develop at the same rate or feel the same, so don't be alarmed if you haven't experienced or noticed certain changes by the date given here.

Each month there is usually something else you need to be thinking about, such as booking your antenatal classes, starting to do special exercises, and buying maternity clothes and nursing bras. These are pointed out at the relevant time in the pregnancy calendar but are covered in greater detail in later chapters.

Becoming pregnant

SIGNS OF PREGNANCY

If you are planning a pregnancy and miss your period, you may suspect that you are pregnant. You may not notice any other changes apart from the missed period at first, but an increase in hormonal activity will confirm your pregnancy with one or more of the following physical signs:
- feeling of nausea at any time
- change in taste: perhaps you will suddenly not be able to tolerate alcohol or coffee
- a preference for certain foods, sometimes close to a craving
- a metallic taste in your mouth
- changes in your breasts; they may feel tender and tingly
- a need to urinate more frequently
- tiredness at any time of the day; you may even feel faint or dizzy too
- increase in normal vaginal discharge
- your emotions swing unpredictably.

DURATION OF PREGNANCY

Pregnancy lasts 266 days from the moment the egg is fertilized. However, actual fertilization is usually difficult to pinpoint precisely. When estimating how pregnant you are, day one of your pregnancy is taken from the first day of your last menstrual period (LMP) and not the day of fertilization. If you have an average 28-day cycle, fertilization is counted as having taken place around day 14 and not day one of your pregnancy. This is because ovulation usually takes place about 14 days before the start of your period.

The pregnancy timescale is thus 266 days plus 14 days – that is, 40 weeks. However, this is only a guide. The average normal pregnancy can last anything from 38 to 42 weeks. You can calculate your estimated date of delivery (EDD) by looking at the table on p. 21.

Weeks 6–10

By this stage of your pregnancy the uterus, which is usually the size and shape of a small pear, has become swollen and slightly enlarged, although it cannot yet be felt above the pubic bone. Visit your doctor to confirm the pregnancy and have a preliminary discussion about the type of birth you wish to have (Chapter 2). You can also arrange what sort of antenatal care you will receive, where, and how to book in (Chapter 3), although booking won't be done until between 10 and 12 weeks.

CONFIRMING PREGNANCY

The pregnancy hormone human chorionic gonadotrophin (HCG) can be detected in tiny amounts in urine. Home kits, available from chemists, are 95 per cent accurate and can confirm a pregnancy within a few days of your missed period.

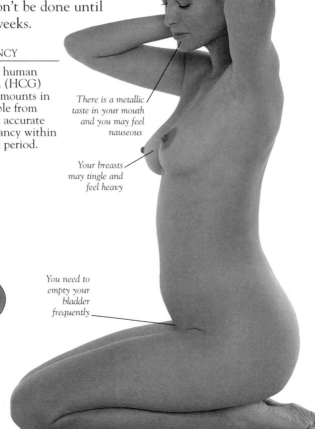

There is a metallic taste in your mouth and you may feel nauseous

Your breasts may tingle and feel heavy

You need to empty your bladder frequently

BABY'S APPEARANCE
AT 8 WEEKS
Length: 25 mm (1 in)
Weight: 3 g (⅒ oz)

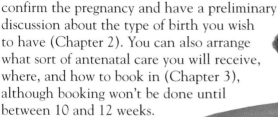

The fetus has a face with a nose, mouth and tongue

The heart and other internal organs are now established

YOUR APPEARANCE
AT 8 WEEKS

Week 12

After about 12 weeks of pregnancy, the irritation of complaints such as morning sickness and frequency of urination should have eased. You may notice a gain in weight for the first time. The amount of blood in your body increases steadily from now on so your heart and lungs have to work harder. Kidneys increase their work too. You may experience some constipation as the bowel slows down. Keep up your normal fitness routine after first checking with your doctor. Book a dental appointment for free NHS treatment.

You feel more stable as your fluctuating hormones begin to settle down

Baby's development

The genital organs can now be seen clearly with ultrasound. The eyes are completely formed and the fingers and toes are developing, though they are still joined by webs of skin. Most of the internal organs are now working. The baby's movements are becoming stronger because his muscles are developing.

Baby's appearance at 12 weeks
Length: 7.5 cm (3 in)
Weight: 18 g (⅝ oz)

Fingers and toes are developing rapidly

You may be able to feel the top of the uterus just above your pubic bone

Earlobes and eyelids are fully formed

Your appearance at 12 weeks

10

Week 16

Y ou will start to feel better and more energetic. You will probably be noticeably pregnant now. Your muscles and ligaments begin to slacken and your waistline disappears. Choose your food carefully; your appetite will increase, and weight gain can be rapid. Start wearing unrestricting clothes (see p. 96) and buy a good bra with adequate support (see p. 97).

MEDICAL TESTS

● A screening blood test may be offered at 15 to 18 weeks to determine your risk of having a baby with Down's syndrome or spina bifida. The substances checked are alpha-fetoprotein (AFP), oestriol and human chorionic gonadotrophin (HCG).
● Higher-than-normal AFP levels could indicate a neural tube defect but can also be caused by a twin pregnancy or by the pregnancy being further advanced than previously thought. Lower-than-normal levels can indicate the risk of Down's syndrome, but further tests will be offered before a definite diagnosis can be made.

BABY'S APPEARANCE AT 16 WEEKS
Length: 16 cm (6 in)
Weight: 135 g (4 ¼ oz)

The skin is transparent

Tiny fingernails are visible

The head appears large for the body

Your hair becomes thicker

The nipples and areola become darker

Your waistline has disappeared and there is a visible bump

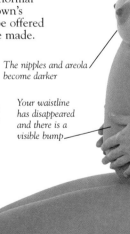

YOUR APPEARANCE AT 16 WEEKS

Week 20

By now you can feel your baby's movements as light, butterfly-like ripples. You'll probably have an ultrasound scan at weeks 20–22, to check your baby's growth. It will also show if there is more than one baby. You should receive your maternity certificate (Form MAT B1) from your doctor or midwife. This entitles you to apply for statutory maternity pay or a weekly maternity allowance (see p. 152).

CHANGES TO YOUR BODY

You start to notice your baby's movements, which are felt as light flutters. Your breasts may produce colostrum, the first milk, and your gums may bleed. You may also experience nasal congestion. Some women have heavy vaginal discharge; if so, use a sanitary pad not a tampon.

BABY'S DEVELOPMENT

The baby's teeth are forming in the jawbone, and he is beginning to move about in the womb.

BABY'S APPEARANCE AT 20 WEEKS
Length: 25 cm (10 in)
Weight: 340 g (12 oz)

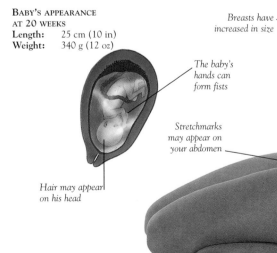

Skin may darken in patches

Breasts have increased in size

The baby's hands can form fists

Stretchmarks may appear on your abdomen

Hair may appear on his head

YOUR APPEARANCE AT 20 WEEKS

Week 24

Your most rapid weight gain takes place around now; your feet will start to feel the strain and you should be conscious of your posture (see p. 80). Wear comfortable shoes and rest with your feet up when possible. By now your heart and lungs are doing 50 per cent more work. Increased fluid levels may cause you to feel hot and sweat more. Your face will look flushed due to increased blood circulation. If born now, your baby would be considered legally viable and could survive with care in a neonatal intensive care unit.

WEIGHT GAIN

You need to gain weight during pregnancy. Gone are the days when weight was watched obsessively and expectant mothers were admonished if they gained too much. The most rapid weight gain is usually between weeks 24 and 32. If you already feel heavy, this is not the time to try to diet. Eat a balanced variety of nutritious and fresh foods instead.

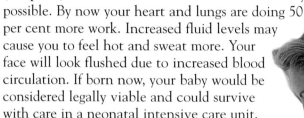

Your face may look puffy because of water retention

BABY'S APPEARANCE AT 24 WEEKS
Length: 33 cm (13 in)
Weight: 570 g (1 ¼ lb)

Increased circulation may cause you to sweat more

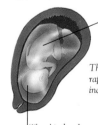

The body is now more in proportion to the head

The bump is enlarging rapidly as the baby increases in size

The skin has lost its translucent quality

YOUR APPEARANCE
AT 24 WEEKS

Week 28

You should tell your employer in writing when you plan to stop work (give three weeks' notice); when the baby is due; and when you intend to return to work. Your antenatal checks may increase to every two to three weeks. If born now, your baby has a more than 50 per cent chance of survival if cared for in an appropriate unit. A second blood test is usually done at 28 weeks to exclude anaemia, which may develop, to check for blood group (rhesus) antibodies and (in some units) to screen for diabetes.

PREGNANCY COMPLAINTS

Approach any minor discomforts of pregnancy sensibly and be assured they will disappear after the birth. If indigestion troubles you, eat little and often and avoid problem foods. If you have cramps, keep up your calcium intake with dairy products.

The veins on your breasts become noticeable

BABY'S APPEARANCE AT 28 WEEKS
Length: 37 cm (14 ½ in)
Weight: 900 g (2 lb)

The womb has risen halfway between your navel and breastbone

He has less room to move and wriggles if you are in a position that he doesn't like

His lungs are now fully developed

YOUR APPEARANCE AT 28 WEEKS

Week 32

If you exert yourself too much you will feel exhausted and breathless. You are probably looking forward to stopping work and should try to rest during the day if possible, especially if you aren't sleeping well. Parentcraft classes will begin soon and you can prepare yourself by gathering all the necessary items for the birth (see p. 112) and perhaps go shopping for the baby too. You may have another blood test to check that you aren't anaemic and that there aren't any rhesus problems (see p. 45).

GOOD POSTURE

Stresses and strains are put on all your joints and ligaments during pregnancy. The change in your centre of gravity as the uterus enlarges can cause unnecessary back pain if you don't watch your posture.

BABY'S APPEARANCE AT 32 WEEKS
Length: 40.5 cm (16 in)
Weight: 1.6 kg (3 ½ lb)

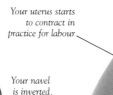

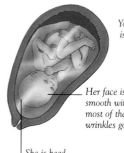

Your uterus starts to contract in practice for labour

Your navel is inverted

Her face is now smooth with most of the wrinkles gone

She is head downwards in the uterus

YOUR APPEARANCE AT 32 WEEKS

Week 36

By now you should be planning your life carefully; don't organize too much activity, instead take on gentle pastimes. Get others to do the running around. Strong Braxton Hicks contractions may make you believe you are in labour (see p. 117). Practise your breathing techniques with the Braxton Hicks.

Antenatal clinics will be at least fortnightly until delivery. For a first baby, the head will "engage" – drop into the pelvic cavity; this eases breathing problems but pain may be felt in the pelvic region. Avoid standing as your ankles might swell. If you have a heavy vaginal discharge, wear light stick-on sanitary pads (never tampons).

BABY'S DEVELOPMENT

The baby is steadily putting on weight. He may now have lots of hair and his fingernails have grown to reach the end of his fingers. The irises of his eyes are blue.

You may have backache and stiff joints

His body is plump and round

Pelvic pain may increase with the pressure of the baby's head

He has shed most of the fine hair (lanugo)

BABY'S APPEARANCE AT 36 WEEKS
Length: 46 cm (18 in)
Weight: 2.5 kg (5 ½ lb)

YOUR APPEARANCE AT 36 WEEKS

Week 40

The expected date of delivery is near and you may become anxious when it passes. Don't worry, however, as only five per cent of babies arrive on the due date. You will be feeling very heavy and tired; all your movements will be an effort and, as the baby is lying deep in your pelvis, you may have pain in the groin and pins and needles down your legs. The baby's movements decrease in force (although not in frequency) because there is less space for her in the uterus. Most babies lie head down ready for birth.

SIGNS OF LABOUR

• a leakage of amniotic fluid; it may be a gush or just a trickle.
• contractions occurring at regular intervals.

Your skin feels tight and itchy

Most of the vernix has gone, but some may still be present in skin folds

Her fingernails are long and she may have scratched herself

Your cervix is softening in preparation for labour

You may have pins and needles

BABY'S APPEARANCE AT 40 WEEKS
Length: 51 cm (20 in)
Weight: 3.4 kg (7½ lb)

YOUR APPEARANCE AT 40 WEEKS

1

Finding out you are pregnant

There are two quite separate aspects to finding out you're pregnant. The first is about confirming your pregnancy; this can be picked up in signs from your body like nausea, having to empty your bladder more often, and dilated veins on the surface of your breasts. The other involves intellectual and emotional acceptance of your pregnancy. The first may be tinged with excitement; the second coloured by feelings of ambivalence. No matter how much you've wanted to be pregnant, you may well have a mixed response to the news that you are.

A mixture of positive and negative feelings about the pregnancy is normal and nothing to feel guilty about. Uppermost in your mind will be your feelings about yourself, your partner and your relationship. Many couples find they reassess each other before accepting their new status. Eventually you'll find that becoming parents is a step forward which introduces you to a satisfying new role.

Early symptoms of pregnancy

PERHAPS THE EARLIEST symptom of pregnancy for many women is the feeling that they really are pregnant – a definite consciousness of pregnancy that I believe has as much to do with the first secretion of pregnancy hormones as anything else. These hormones affect your body in every respect, as well as your mind and the way you feel.

Another early sign is fatigue. Although some women feel energized, the majority would confess to feeling tired. It is a new

kind of tiredness that they haven't felt before. Some women say that they find themselves dropping off to sleep at any time of the day; others say that they become so sleepy in the early afternoon that they have to stop what they are doing and wait for the tiredness to pass. Others are tired in the evening. Whenever it occurs, this fatigue is often uncontrollable and you just have to sleep. This condition is known as narcolepsy. I have never found a satisfactory explanation for this eccentric desire to sleep. It could well be an effect of progesterone, which reaches high levels in the blood early in pregnancy. Progesterone is a sedative in human beings with powerful tranquillizing and hypnotic effects. Progesterone also accounts for the serene and beatific look that is classically associated with pregnancy. There is another type of fatigue, occurring later in pregnancy, which is due simply to tiredness of the body, but it rarely occurs during the first three months.

MISSED PERIOD

Within two weeks of fertilization you'll miss a period – the classic sign of pregnancy. This is called amenorrhoea. While pregnancy is the commonest cause of amenorrhoea, it's not the only one so don't automatically assume you're pregnant. A severe physical illness, shock, jet lag, surgery, even anxiety, are known to make a period late. Equally, it's quite common to have a light bleed after the pregnancy is established, at the time you might normally have had a period. This is why some pregnancies appear only to be eight months in length (see p. 55).

MORNING SICKNESS

Nausea, occasionally accompanied by vomiting, occurs from about week six and is often experienced as "morning sickness", though it may happen at other times of the day. It rarely continues beyond the first three months and then it gradually stops. It's caused by the increasing levels of hormones circulating in the blood, which can have a direct irritant effect on the lining of the stomach. One hormone, human chorionic gonadotrophin (HCG), is produced to keep up supplies of oestrogen and progesterone to maintain the pregnancy. Its presence in urine confirms a pregnancy (see p. 20). The build-up of HCG roughly parallels the time of nausea, tailing off at

12–14 weeks. Hormones also cause a rapid clearing of sugar from the blood, which may result in a simultaneous feeling of hunger and sickness.

TASTES AND CRAVINGS

A change in taste and in preferences for certain foods may be one of the first signs of pregnancy, happening even before you miss a period. It's quite common to go off certain food and drink, especially fried foods, coffee and alcohol. Some women experience a metallic taste in the mouth which affects their appreciation of food. Cravings are thought to be due to the rising hormone levels and are sometimes felt during the second half of the menstrual cycle for the same reason. Don't indulge a craving for high calorie foods, which may be low in nutritional value.

FREQUENCY OF URINATION

As the uterus begins to swell, it presses on the bladder. Hormonal changes lead to differences in muscle tone, also affecting the bladder. As a result, it tries to expel even small amounts of urine, and many women notice a desire to pass urine more frequently only a week after conception. Unless there's a burning sensation or pain when you pass urine there is no need to consult your doctor about frequency of urination (micturition). Around week 12, the enlarging uterus rises up out of the pelvic cavity which reduces the pressure on the bladder for the next few months.

BREASTS

The breast changes in early pregnancy (see p. 56) are due to stimulation by progesterone. Even before you miss your first period your nipples will feel sore and your breasts will enlarge and become tender. Veins are prominent over the surface of the breasts and the creamy nodules in the nipple area (the areola) will become bigger. The nipples also start to enlarge and deepen in colour.

Receiving the news

MOST OF US FEEL some ambivalence about pregnancy and parenthood and find that our feelings shift with our moods. It's absolutely normal to have mixed feelings. It would be unrealistic to imagine that your life will remain unchanged after the baby comes and it's better to think ahead. Don't feel that you're inadequate for having conflicting feelings and don't try to suppress them. It's far more sensible to acknowledge and face up to them, rather than trying to reach a point where there are no conflicts. Going through pregnancy is a phase of your emotional growth, and at the end of it you should have a better understanding and awareness of yourself.

PREGNANCY TESTS

There are various ways to confirm pregnancy. Detecting the presence of the pregnancy hormone human chorionic gonadotrophin (see p. 56) in urine is the most common test. This hormone is produced in increasing amounts in the early part of pregnancy.

Home kits
Finding out whether you are pregnant in the privacy of your home may help to ease any feelings of nervousness you have and you can be sure of complete confidentiality. Home pregnancy testing kits are at least 90 per cent reliable, though they are quite expensive. They can be used from the day your period is due, but the result will be more certain if you wait for another couple of days. Positive results are rarely wrong, but false negatives may occur if the test is used too early.

The kits use a urine sample and it is essential to follow the instructions on the packet exactly, since methods vary from kit to kit. Read through them carefully before you start. It is also very important that you use the first urine you pass after waking in the morning. The pregnancy hormone will be in its most concentrated form at this time, since you haven't eaten or drunk anything for a number of hours.

Urine tests
Pass a sample of your first urine of the morning into a clean, soap-free container. Your doctor, clinic or chemist will arrange for the test to be done. A negative result from a urine test does not necessarily mean you are not pregnant. If the other signs persist, try again in seven days; you may have tested too early in your pregnancy. Laboratory urine tests are 95 per cent reliable.

Unexpected results
It is possible that a test will show a positive result that becomes negative when repeated, and your period may start a few days later. Don't worry. Half of all conceptions do not become established pregnancies, as the fertilized egg fails to implant in the lining of the uterus and there is a natural termination. The test may have been positive because it was done before the loss of the fertilized egg. To avoid this error, do the test around the time of your first missed period. If there is a weak but positive result, repeat the test a few days later with a fresh sample.

Do you have the right result?
A number of factors can affect whether your pregnancy test results are accurate.
● In older women, hormonal changes caused by approaching menopause can give false positives or negatives.
● Incorrectly collected or stored urine can lead to errors.
● If the test is performed too early, the concentration of human chorionic gonadotrophin (HCG) will be too low to detect. It is important to know when your period was due. Irregular or infrequent periods can affect an accurate indication of pregnancy.
● Antidepressant or fertility drugs containing HCG can change the results. Contraceptive pills, antibiotics and painkillers should not have any effect.
● If the equipment used for the test is too hot, the result may be false. Urine must be room temperature at the time of the test.

DIFFERENT REACTIONS

The reactions to the confirmation of your pregnancy may not be what you expected. It's possible that personal circumstances change so that a pregnancy is unwelcome. A woman may resent a pregnancy taking over her body and become bitter because her active life is curtailed. Some women become depressed when they realize they are pregnant and even consider abortion.

This is painting a negative picture, more negative perhaps than the majority of women feel. However, the most important part of receiving the news that you're pregnant is for you and your partner to accept the pregnancy fully. Don't think that you can ignore it and carry on as normal just because it doesn't show for the first few weeks or months. You both have to think of your pregnancy realistically, not in a rosy glow.

HOW TO CALCULATE YOUR ESTIMATED DATE OF DELIVERY (EDD)

The average pregnancy is 266 days long measured from conception or 280 days measured from the first day of your last menstrual period (LMP). To find your EDD, find the date of your LMP in the columns of dates set in bold type; the date next to it is your EDD. You can also work it out as follows:

LMP 17.09.03
+ 9 months 17.06.04
+ 7 days 24.06.04

Remember 280 days is average and you may not be average. The possibility of your baby arriving on your EDD depends on your having regular 28-day cycles. All that doctors are prepared to say is that a normal pregnancy may be anywhere between 38 and 42 weeks.

Jan	Oct	Feb	Nov	Mar	Dec	Apr	Jan	May	Feb	June	Mar	July	Apr	Aug	May	Sept	June	Oct	July	Nov	Aug	Dec	Sept
1	8	1	8	1	6	1	6	1	5	1	8	1	7	1	8	1	8	1	8	1	8	1	7
2	9	2	9	2	7	2	7	2	6	2	9	2	8	2	9	2	9	2	9	2	9	2	8
3	10	3	10	3	8	3	8	3	7	3	10	3	9	3	10	3	10	3	10	3	10	3	9
4	11	4	11	4	9	4	9	4	8	4	11	4	10	4	11	4	11	4	11	4	11	4	10
5	12	5	12	5	10	5	10	5	9	5	12	5	11	5	12	5	12	5	12	5	12	5	11
6	13	6	13	6	11	6	11	6	10	6	13	6	12	6	13	6	13	6	13	6	13	6	12
7	14	7	14	7	12	7	12	7	11	7	14	7	13	7	14	7	14	7	14	7	14	7	13
8	15	8	15	8	13	8	13	8	12	8	15	8	14	8	15	8	15	8	15	8	15	8	14
9	16	9	16	9	14	9	14	9	13	9	16	9	15	9	16	9	16	9	16	9	16	9	15
10	17	10	17	10	15	10	15	10	14	10	17	10	16	10	17	10	17	10	17	10	17	10	16
11	18	11	18	11	16	11	16	11	15	11	18	11	17	11	18	11	18	11	18	11	18	11	17
12	19	12	19	12	17	12	17	12	16	12	19	12	18	12	19	12	19	12	19	12	19	12	18
13	20	13	20	13	18	13	18	13	17	13	20	13	19	13	20	13	20	13	20	13	20	13	19
14	21	14	21	14	19	14	19	14	18	14	21	14	20	14	21	14	21	14	21	14	21	14	20
15	22	15	22	15	20	15	20	15	19	15	22	15	21	15	22	15	22	15	22	15	22	15	21
16	23	16	23	16	21	16	21	16	20	16	23	16	22	16	23	16	23	16	23	16	23	16	22
17	24	17	24	17	22	17	22	17	21	17	24	17	23	17	24	17	24	17	24	17	24	17	23
18	25	18	25	18	23	18	23	18	22	18	25	18	24	18	25	18	25	18	25	18	25	18	24
19	26	19	26	19	24	19	24	19	23	19	26	19	25	19	26	19	26	19	26	19	26	19	25
20	27	20	27	20	25	20	25	20	24	20	27	20	26	20	27	20	27	20	27	20	27	20	26
21	28	21	28	21	26	21	26	21	25	21	28	21	27	21	28	21	28	21	28	21	28	21	27
22	29	22	29	22	27	22	27	22	26	22	29	22	28	22	29	22	29	22	29	22	29	22	28
23	30	23	30	23	28	23	28	23	27	23	30	23	29	23	30	23	30	23	30	23	30	23	29
24	31	24	1	24	29	24	29	24	28	24	31	24	30	24	31	24	1	24	31	24	31	24	30
25	1	25	2	25	30	25	30	25	1	25	1	25	1	25	1	25	1	25	1	25	1	25	1
26	2	26	3	26	31	26	31	26	2	26	2	26	2	26	2	26	3	26	2	26	2	26	2
27	3	27	4	27	1	27	1	27	3	27	3	27	3	27	3	27	4	27	3	27	3	27	3
28	4	28	5	28	2	28	2	28	4	28	4	28	4	28	4	28	5	28	4	28	4	28	4
29	5			29	3	29	3	29	5	29	5	29	5	29	5	29	6	29	5	29	5	29	5
30	6			30	4	30	4	30	6	30	6	30	6	30	6	30	7	30	6	30	6	30	6
31	7			31	5			31	7			31	7	31	7			31	7			31	7

Jan	Nov	Feb	Dec	Mar	Jan	Apr	Feb	May	Mar	June	Apr	July	May	Aug	June	Sept	July	Oct	Aug	Nov	Sept	Dec	Oct

The working woman

IN MOST COUNTRIES there are laws governing the length of time that a woman has to work in order to receive financial benefits (see p. 152) and the conditions that her employer must meet on her return to work. Outside these laws the majority of employers are keen to cooperate with your plans for discontinuing employment before the birth and for resuming it afterwards. There is usually a statutory period of notice of maternity leave that you must give your employer; if you don't comply with this you may lose benefits, so find out about your rights as early in the pregnancy as possible. Around the end of the first trimester you should be thinking about your future work. If you wish to have your job held open for you after your maternity leave, talk to your employer to see how your plans can be accommodated.

WORKING DURING PREGNANCY

Unless your work involves heavy physical labour, or you work in an environment where there are harmful chemicals or fumes, there is no reason why you should not continue

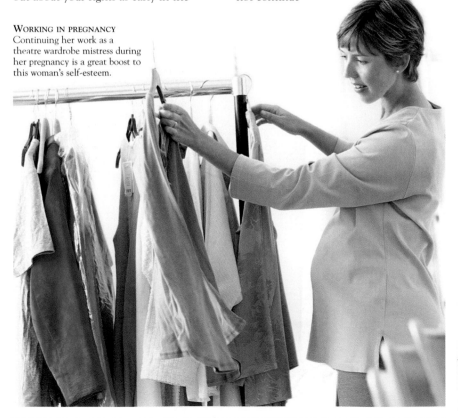

WORKING IN PREGNANCY
Continuing her work as a theatre wardrobe mistress during her pregnancy is a great boost to this woman's self-esteem.

working well into pregnancy. The length of time that you will work depends on your physical fitness, the sort of job you are doing and your reason for working. One benefit of working is that it encourages everyone around you to view pregnancy as normal. As well as that, your job gives you a feeling of tability and security during a time when you are undergoing physical and psychological changes.

There's no hard and fast rule about when to give up work – it depends on the nature of the work you do and how physically taxing it is. Probably 32 weeks is a good time to stop as it is around this time that the greatest work load is thrown

on your heart, lungs and other vital organs like the kidneys and liver, and there is a great deal of physical stress on your spine, your joints and muscles. It is a time when you should not be asking your body to do anything except rest if you feel tired. This is difficult in a job, even a sedentary one.

Whatever your job, you will have to make adjustments to your daily routine. In later pregnancy, you will lose some of your agility, and working long hours and having late nights will leave you exhausted. You will find yourself falling asleep and losing concentration. As far as household chores are concerned, let your priorities slide. Your health and that of your unborn baby are far more important than a spotless house.

TIPS FOR THE WORKING DAY

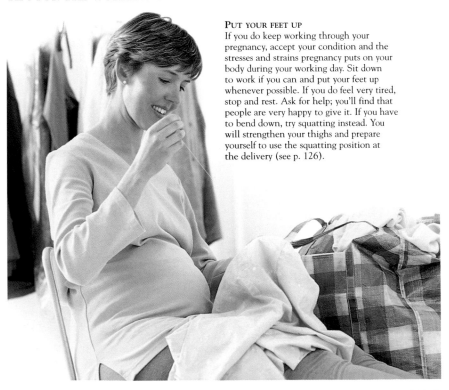

PUT YOUR FEET UP
If you do keep working through your pregnancy, accept your condition and the stresses and strains pregnancy puts on your body during your working day. Sit down to work if you can and put your feet up whenever possible. If you do feel very tired, stop and rest. Ask for help; you'll find that people are very happy to give it. If you have to bend down, try squatting instead. You will strengthen your thighs and prepare yourself to use the squatting position at the delivery (see p. 126).

BEING A WORKING MOTHER

Some women are happy to deal with pregnancy as an interruption to their work, remaining in their posts until just before going into labour, then having the baby and returning to work within the shortest time possible. They avoid the emotional dilemma of whether or not to breast or bottle feed the baby and opt for the latter. Other women would be unhappy with this decision. They want to stay with their children; anything that takes them away from their children is painful.

Women with strong maternal instincts will be concerned with not only depriving their babies of affection, but also with the sacrifices that they are making themselves. They want to enjoy their children's presence and company much of the time, and, especially while their children are young, find it distressing to leave them even for a few hours.

Nonetheless, mothers continue to work for many different reasons, which include economic necessity, the desire to be independent and self-reliant, boredom with the routine of home life, and the absolute personal need to work. As women become more able to shape their own lives, more mothers are working, and of these more and more do so simply because they enjoy it. They feel that their work greatly enriches their lives and that if it does, that will certainly help to enrich their family life.

In the past, many women thought it was their duty to ignore their own desires and serve the family; now most women feel very strongly that they have the right to take their own wishes into consideration and to make the decision to work, even if they know that it may create difficulties in the family.

Your partner's feelings should also be considered along with your own. It can lead only to unhappiness and resentment if you decide to return to work but your partner is reluctant for you to do so. If you have reason to believe that he feels this way, you must bring matters out into the open. A frank discussion with him may lead to a suitable compromise and a happy solution to your working future.

WHEN TO RETURN

If you decide that you are going to return to work after your baby is born, you might want to go back under different conditions. Discuss this with your employer during your pregnancy. There may be provision for part-time employment in your work or a phased return which allows you to be in effect a part-time worker up until one year after the baby's birth. You might like to investigate job-sharing or setting up on your own in some freelance activity, which might enable you to work from home. Now is the time to think about these alternatives and plan for them.

In figuring out when you are going to restart work, you must be fair to yourself. It takes about nine months for your metabolism to return to normal after a pregnancy; parts of your body recover more quickly than others. If you menstruate three months after giving birth, this is a good sign that your ovaries are getting back to their normal cyclical routine, but not all your hormone glands will be in step with them. The muscles, ligaments and joints become more flexible and elastic to accommodate your pregnant shape and weight and need time to regain their tone and strength after the birth. Vital organs like the heart, kidneys and lungs, and your blood, gradually adjust to coping with you alone and not with you plus the baby.

BABIES AND PARENTS

A good system of childcare will be a priority and you'll have to put quite a lot of time and effort into selecting one that suits your needs. If you feel reluctant or guilty about entrusting your baby to someone else, and fear that you might be left out of your child's affections, be reassured as I was (even though only in

ADVANTAGES AND DISADVANTAGES OF BEING A WORKING MOTHER

ADVANTAGES

- increased independence
- financial rewards – the chance to raise the standard of living of your family
- career fulfilment – chance to use whatever training and qualifications you may have
- more intense interaction with your child when you are at home
- intellectual need to work – bored and lonely at home
- ability to maintain a high profile in your chosen field.

DISADVANTAGES

- sense of guilt and inadequacy because you feel you are neglecting your child
- isolation from the community
- tiredness because you are juggling two jobs at once
- great stress due to dual responsibilities and the need to be constantly planning ahead
- resentment of full-time mothers in your community
- worries about finding and keeping good child care.

retrospect) by an interesting study carried out in the last few years. When I actually was a working mother with small babies, I didn't know that this research was going on and trusted my own instinct. What I felt was that my children would know me as their mother by the biological semaphore that I sent out and that they picked up. I felt certain in my own mind, despite the presence of very loving nannies, that my children could never mistake a nanny for me, their mother. I found it difficult to pin down how they would make the distinction. I thought possibly that it would be through body smell and until they were about 18 months I made sure that they had opportunities to feel and smell my skin at feeding times and during nuzzling play.

What research showed was that babies have an even keener intelligence for singling out their parents from all other human beings than I thought. The crucial factor is the loving, interested attention that only parents can give, and a baby sorts this out from all the other stimuli. The most staggering aspect of this research is that babies need less than an hour a day of caring parental interest to thrive. The length of time spent without their parents counts far less than the quality of the time spent with them. Love isn't measured in time, love is what you put into time, no matter how short.

DUAL ROLE

Having to invest most of your free time in your family can be hard for a working mother. There's no denying that you are doing two jobs. Sometimes this is not too difficult. If you have an office job, you may have the energy to spare when you get home for bathtimes, play, story reading and sympathetic listening. However, a physical job or any job that involves caring or communication, means expending much of the sort of energy your children need during your working day.

I firmly believe that a child, especially of pre-school age, has the right to expect and receive his parents' attention when they are home from work. The price of this is high. Instead of dropping into a chair or soaking in a bath when you return home, you'll have to pick up the baby and do everything else one-handed until he's asleep. When you finally fall asleep, ten to one your night will be disturbed. You don't just have to be generous of spirit, you both have to be sacrificial. There are advantages and disadvantages to being a working mother (see above); the best option for you is whatever makes you happiest. Be prepared, however, for feelings of guilt and inadequacy, but so long as you and your partner are happy, your child will do equally well whether you stay at home or go to work.

2

Choices in childbirth

Most women are aware that there are choices to be made in childbirth and, given a normal pregnancy, they can exercise many personal options. In most parts of the UK, doctors and midwives form flexible teams that work towards satisfying a woman's birth preferences. You can now feel that the birth of your child is an experience over which you have control and which you are free to enjoy. Hospitals welcome the presence of your partner or someone else close to you as a birth attendant. Home births are also becoming more common and with the advent of the team midwife scheme, a doctor need no longer be present at a home birth unless complications occur.

Organizing yourself

SOME WOMEN ARE disappointed by their experience of childbirth; not the birth itself but the way it's conducted or the way they're treated. If you're going to have the kind of birth you want, you need to be explicit in stating your desires. Second, you have to be aware of your options. The way you can achieve this is by reading, asking questions, writing to various associations for information and guidance (see pp. 154–155), being somewhat more self-assertive than you might have been in the past and never accepting anything unless you feel entirely happy about it. Third, you are going to have to learn to communicate. It's all very well having decided in your own head what you would like to happen

but if you can't explain this to others your hopes will never be realized. Set things out on paper in a logical way so that they are clear in your own mind. If you haven't a lot of self-confidence, ask your partner or a good friend to come along for moral support when you have to face a situation that makes you anxious.

One aim of this chapter is to make it easy for you to plan the kind of childbirth you would like after assessing your own emotional and physical needs. Another aim is to give you the confidence to discuss with doctors and midwives on equal terms the options available and to state your preferences. Most hospital notes have a page for you to record your birth plan so that your wishes are available for all to see.

WHERE TO HAVE YOUR BABY

The two important elements in your choice are whether you want a medically managed or a natural childbirth and whether you want to have your baby at home or in hospital. There are people who passionately advocate hospital high-technology births, who say that this is the only way to ensure that mother and baby will be well looked after, if an emergency occurs. At the other extreme, there are natural childbirth advocates who are vehement in support of their methods. Some women feel that only in hospital will they have the security they need. Other women wish to be surrounded by hearth and home when they give birth to their baby. You should consider the following options.

Consultant maternity unit

This is obstetrician-based care within a general hospital. Most antenatal care is done in the community; however, women who may have complications attend the antenatal clinic at the hospital. In this case you may well be seen by different doctors and midwives at each visit, though now many hospitals have introduced team midwives. Some centres across the country now have birthing pools and other facilities so a woman can have the labour she prefers. For first-time mothers the support of other mothers and hospital staff during the first days is an advantage, although a busy hospital may not be restful for some. The emphasis in a hospital maternity unit will be on helping you to have a normal birth. However, it is here that you are more likely to experience so-called "high-tech" obstetric procedures, which are available if necessary.

Domino scheme

A district midwife from a local team looks after you antenatally in partnership with your own family doctor. When you go into labour, your regular midwife, or one who is on call at the time, will take you to hospital and deliver you there. You can go home with your midwife within six hours of the birth if all is going well, and you're unlikely to be in hospital more than 48 hours.

At home

At one time medical opinion was almost 100 per cent of the view that hospital delivery was safer than a home birth. However, studies have shown that women are much happier at home and it has been proved that it is at least as safe to give birth at home as in hospital for a healthy mother and her baby. Most midwives will agree to a home birth if they feel it is safe for the mother.

General practitioner unit

These are only available in some areas. Your doctor and a midwife look after your antenatal and postnatal care. Either the midwife or your doctor will deliver you in the unit within a hospital where the atmosphere is much less rushed than in a large maternity hospital.

GETTING INFORMATION

Like any other expectant animal, spend some time finding out where and how you are going to have the baby. One of the first things to do is to talk to your doctor. He or she will give you information about what is available and the various people that you might get in touch with. Your doctor will also tell you the kind of birth he or she prefers and you'll be able to assess if you're going to get on easily or if there may be conflict. This will help you to make a decision. At the same time contact your midwife. More and more women are opting for midwife-supervised births; and while it's always advisable to work with your doctor, most recognize now that a normal birth can be handled perfectly safely by a trained midwife. Your midwife will give you the addresses of the various associations to write to.

Home birth

THERE ARE ADVANTAGES to having
your baby at home if your pregnancy is
straightforward. You'll avoid exhausting
travel to hospital when you're already in
labour, and you'll have the same midwife
throughout labour and birth. Starting off
breastfeeding is nearly always more
successful in the home environment. The
other important factor is that you lead the
way in managing your labour and birth;
others support you.

MOBILITY

Mobility is now recognized as being
positively helpful during labour. Most
women find it easier to cope with
contractions if they are able to change
position at will; it also helps the uterus to
work better and keeps the oxygen to the
baby topped up. Although hospitals
encourage mobility, many women prefer
to have the freedom and privacy of
moving about in their own home.

CONFIDENCE

You'll probably feel confident and relaxed
because you're in a familiar place. This is
a great advantage, as emotional well-being
does affect the function of the uterus.
You'll also avoid the possibility of cross-
infection from the medical staff and other
mothers and babies in hospital. Being at
home will avoid many aspects of hospital
care that you may find distasteful. Their
absence will be a bonus.

FAMILIAR SURROUNDINGS
After a home birth, you will both feel more relaxed
as you are in your own familiar surroundings.

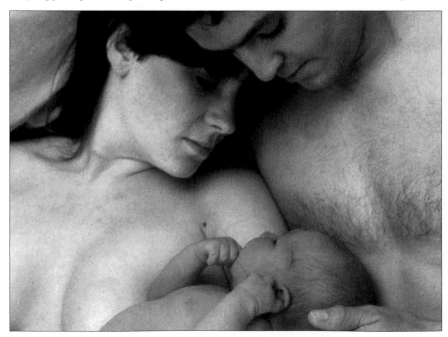

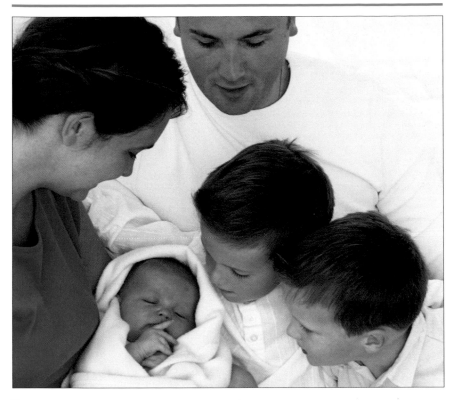

FAMILY GROUP

By staying at home you'll avoid unhappiness caused by family separation, particularly if you have other children. Everyone can benefit from the emotional and physical bonding that develops immediately after the birth (see p. 148).

ORGANIZING A HOME BIRTH

The first step is to consult your doctor and ask if you can have maternity care from that practice. You may have to find a different doctor to look after you during pregnancy. Some doctors or even whole health authorities are unwilling to authorize home deliveries, especially in rural areas where a specialist maternity unit may be many miles away, resulting

A FAMILY EVENT
If you have your baby at home the whole family will feel involved with the new baby from the start.

in dangerous delay if anything untoward happens during labour or birth. If there isn't a doctor in your area who does home confinements, ring a relevant organization for help and advice (see pp. 154–155).

Provided there have been no problems in your health or during a previous labour, you should find a general practitioner or hospital consultant who will take responsibility for you. Community midwives will then take over your care. They cannot legally refuse to deliver you and after you are assessed by the doctor, you can prepare for your home birth. If you get no satisfaction, write to the Director of Midwifery in your area.

Hospital birth

FOR SOME WOMEN the decision to have a hospital birth is made for them because of their physical condition or their obstetric history. However, if you do need or want a hospital confinement, before you decide on a particular hospital, there are many questions that you may want to ask. Use this checklist to help you.
• Can my partner or friend stay with me during labour and delivery?
• If I need a Caesarean section, can my partner or a friend be with me?

WHY A HOSPITAL DELIVERY?

There are good reasons for having a hospital birth:
• If your medical background includes heart disease, kidney disease, high blood pressure, tuberculosis, asthma, diabetes, serious anaemia, obesity or epilepsy.
• If your previous deliveries have included a stillbirth, breech presentation, a transverse or oblique lie (that is if the baby is lying sideways in the pelvis), premature labour before the 37th week, placental insufficiency where the placenta failed to nourish the baby adequately, a forceps delivery or a retained placenta.
• If the following obstetric reasons apply in your case: the baby is too big to pass through the pelvis; true postmaturity (see p. 141); you have pre-eclampsia; you are carrying twins or higher multiples; you have bleeding from the vagina late in pregnancy; the placenta is lying in the lower part of the uterus (placenta praevia); there is excessive water around the baby; you are a Rhesus negative mother and tests have shown that there are sufficient antibodies in your blood to harm the baby; you have scarring of the uterus from previous Caesarean sections or you are over 35 years old and it is your first baby (although this is no longer necessarily a reason for special attention if you are healthy.

• May I walk around during labour if everything is okay?
• May I choose the position in which I can give birth?
• Do women have their waters broken as a routine?
• What percentage of women do you induce in this hospital?
• How many women have continuous electronic fetal monitoring?
• What percentage of women have an episiotomy or a forceps delivery in this hospital?
• Can I arrange to have no drugs for pain relief in this hospital?
• When a Caesarean birth is planned how many women have epidural anaesthesia and how many have general anaesthesia?
• Can I have as much time as I want to cuddle the baby after delivery if everything is okay?
• If I have a Caesarean section can I and/ or the father hold the baby afterwards?
• Can I use aromatherapy oils during labour for massage?
• Is there free visiting time?
• Is it possible to arrange a six-, 12- or 24-hour discharge?

HOW LONG?

Your hospital stay can be as short as six hours and this is becoming increasingly normal in busy maternity units. A fairly standard stay is 48 hours, and even after a Caesarean you are likely to be discharged after five days provided the incision is healing and the baby is healthy. However, it is your right to discharge yourself from hospital, on your own responsibility, at any time. If you have adequate support and help and there are no complications with you or your baby, there is no reason why you should not go home.

HELPING YOU THROUGH LABOUR
Your partner or a friend can stay with you in hospital to encourage you throughout labour and delivery.

YOUR BIRTH PARTNER

Your partner should be closely involved
in the pregnancy and birth, and he is the
natural choice for a birth assistant. His
involvement is crucial not only as support
for you but also for cementing the bonds
with the baby from the moment of birth.
He can be the most loving and supportive

"midwife". His involvement from
the beginning will improve your
communication in preparation for the
birth, and during labour your partner is
the person who gives you most attention.
The medical staff are there to support the
two of you. However, your birth assistant
doesn't have to be your partner. You may
prefer a relative or close friend instead.

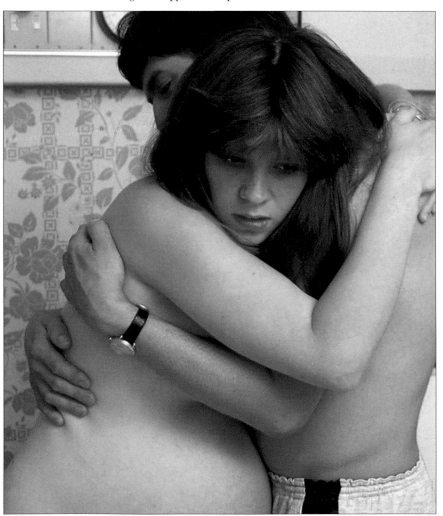

THE MIDWIFE

A midwife-supervised pregnancy and labour guarantees continuity of care, a factor that is missing from many hospital pregnancies. Whenever you attend the antenatal clinic you will see one of the team midwives so you can get to know them all during your pregnancy, and one of the team will attend you during the birth.

THE OBSTETRICIAN

Some women, however, feel cheated and nervous, even second class, if they don't have an obstetrician, as well as a midwife

present at their delivery. Despite the fact that they expect nothing to go wrong, they would simply be happier in the hands of a specialist. There is yet another group of women for whom the hospital setting makes childbirth the event they expect it to be.

As obstetricians usually only attend difficult births and emergencies, you should expect to pay quite a substantial amount for private attendance. Private health care in the UK does not usually

SENSE OF ACHIEVEMENT
After the birth, you will both feel that you have achieved something miraculous together.

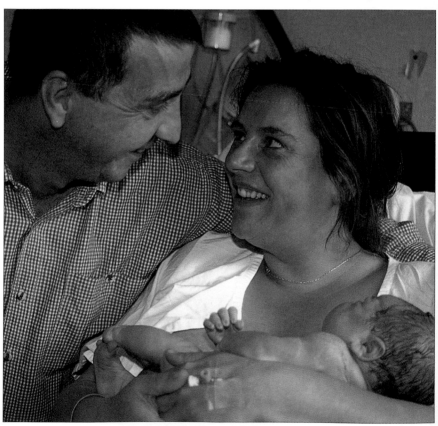

cover antenatal care, or delivery except for Caesarean section. Obstetricians are busy people, and on your day of delivery he or she may not be available. You may not even see the same doctor at the antenatal clinic. If you do want to go privately, get a list of practitioners from the Royal College of Obstetrics and Gynaecology (see p. 155) to help you decide on the right obstetrician for you.

The natural childbirth movement

AS OBSTETRIC MEDICINE became more sophisticated, childbirth gradually came to be seen as a medical condition – something to be overseen by doctors instead of the natural, straightforward process that it really is. However from the 1960s there was a movement by women (helped by midwives) to reclaim natural childbirth. This means giving birth without fear, without unnecessary medical intervention and in a calm atmosphere. Several methods were propounded with slightly differing emphases, some of which centred on the mother, others on the baby, and still others on both. But the net result was a gradual and welcome changing of attitudes so that in the majority of hospitals the best points of the different approaches have been adopted and developed. Originally, however, there was a pure form of each method.

GRANTLY DICK-READ

In his book *Childbirth Without Fear*, first published in the 1940s, Dr Grantly Dick-Read brought the principles of natural childbirth to public attention. His philosophy was to try to lessen and hopefully eliminate fear and tension, and the pain that resulted from these emotions, through proper education and emotional support. The Grantly Dick-Read method taught women how to cope with tension but lay strong emphasis on the fact that knowledge allays fear and prevents tension, which in turn controls pain. To help do this, he developed courses of instruction that included breathing control exercises and relaxation of muscles (see p. 103), information on what to expect in a normal situation and what women can do to help themselves. His method also taught mothers how to look for support in the form of guidance, reassurance and sympathy. Grantly Dick-Read laid great store on preparation for parenthood and childbirth itself.

PSYCHOPROPHYLAXIS

This involves training in breathing methods as a preparation for labour. The techniques were pioneered in Russia and introduced in the West by Dr Fernand Lamaze. The Lamaze method is by far the most popular in the United States and is the basis for the teaching of the National Childbirth Trust in Britain. It encourages the woman to take responsibility for herself, to enter into partnership with her companions, friends and counsellors. It greatly values team work. The woman must prepare her body throughout pregnancy with special exercises and she has to train her mind to respond automatically to each type of contraction she will feel in labour. Her partner acts as "coach" and as emotional support. He is expected to attend the course with the expectant mother and co-operate with her at home on the conditioning exercises, and he coaches, coaxes and comforts her throughout labour and delivery.

THE LEBOYER PHILOSOPHY

This relies on several basic precepts and relates more to the baby than the mother and her progress throughout labour. Dr Frederick Leboyer in his book *Birth Without Violence* states that the newborn baby feels everything, reflecting all the emotions surrounding it – anger, anxiety, impatience and so on – and that the baby is extremely sensitive through its skin, its ears, its eyes. For that reason he believes that all stimulation to the baby should be minimized with low lights, few sounds, little handling, and with immersion in water at body heat so that the baby's entry into the world is as little different from its life in the womb as possible.

This teaching is in fact not entirely in line with the physiology of what occurs at the moment of birth for the baby. It is contact with air at a temperature different from body temperature that makes the baby take its first gulp of air to start the initial crucial function of the lungs and causes the baby's blood circulation to change from a fetal one to a mature one.

It is also simply not true to say that a baby's hearing is so sensitive that it is disturbed by noises around it. The sound of the uterine vessels within the womb are akin to a loud vacuum cleaner. Leboyer also believes that the mother is an "enemy and a monster" to the child, driving it and crushing it within the birth passage. He likens her to a torturer. Many women reasonably object to this view as it minimizes, even diminishes, the role of the mother.

Dr Leboyer believes that the baby should not be touched by foreign materials but by human skin. The ideal place for the baby is to be laid face down on the mother's abdomen and covered by her arms. It has been proven by experiment, not Leboyer's, that this is far more efficient in preventing the baby from losing heat than overhead heaters. Research has shown that the baby is able to clear mucus from its respiratory passages more efficiently when lying face down on its mother's stomach than with a suction tube. Leboyer suggests that the curtains and blinds in the delivery room are drawn and the lights are dimmed. Some medical authorities object to this as they say it is not possible to assess the baby's condition in a dim light.

Few centres practise the pure Leboyer method but many hospitals and community midwives practise Leboyer-based birth. It seemed to me on first reading Leboyer that all he had done was to formalize what midwives had been doing, in principle, for years. Hospitals were slower to adopt Leboyer because research has shown that Leboyer babies appear to receive no extra benefit compared to others, though many "Leboyer mothers" may feel they do.

DR MICHEL ODENT

A French doctor named Michel Odent has advocated placing the mother in an environment which is cosy and home-like, giving her complete freedom to act as she wishes and encouraging her to reach a new level of animal consciousness where she forgets her inhibitions and returns to a rather primitive biological state. Dr Odent believes that the high levels of endorphins, the body's natural narcotics, should be allowed to have full rein in the mother's body. He logically argues that if a woman is given pain-killers and analgesics her endorphins are cut off, thus depriving her of the benefit of natural pain relief.

Dr Odent's clinic in Pithiviers in France, where he pioneered his natural childbirth techniques, became a centre for those who wished to change opinions and practices in childbirth. Dr Odent believes that during labour there should be music, soft furnishings, and a relaxed atmosphere. A woman who goes into labour should be allowed to sit, walk, stand, eat and drink, and do whatever she wants. Women should not be interfered with in any way and can take up whatever position is most comfortable at any stage of the labour. Left to their own devices many women take up a position on all fours which seems to help the pain. Later on in birth many stand up or semi-squat so that the force of gravity can help them, a natural thing to do, which most primitive tribes practise. Odent encourages the supported squatting position where he, or the woman's partner, stands behind her, takes her weight underneath her armpits and upper arms and allows her to bend her knees and place her weight on her partner's arm.

Dr Odent believes that birthing pools, which he now uses for many home water births, should be primarily viewed as a means of pain relief. The birth itself does not need to be underwater, though Dr Odent is quite happy to deliver the baby into the water of the bath if that is what happens. There seems to be no proof that an underwater birth is dangerous to the baby so long as the head is lifted out of the water immediately.

Dr Odent's methods have always had low rates of episiotomy, forceps and Caesarean section. The supported squat position is the one which prevents severe perineal tears during delivery. Because the mother has been in an upright position when the baby emerges she remains sitting upright with the cord still intact and the baby in her lap. The baby immediately smells the mother's skin and it is thought that this is important to the baby in establishing breastfeeding. Within a few seconds most mothers instinctively lift the baby up and place it at the breast. No partner needs to be told to encircle the mother and the baby with his own body and arms. Each will do what comes naturally in these very personal moments.

YOGA-BASED METHODS

This is not just for those who already practise yoga. During birth a woman should concentrate her awareness on being totally at one with what is happening to her. Through yogic methods she is able to control her awareness according to her capacity and tolerance so at some times she is able to distract herself from the contractions and at others be totally involved in them. She may use meditation and chanting with the support of yoga groups' spiritual participation. Practitioners in the yogic methods believe that a woman can handle childbirth in a mature and serene way. Yogic childbirth education helps in the belief that a woman has the ability to create or destroy her own pain and joy during birth.

Nursing and medical procedures

ONE OF THE MOST WELCOME outcomes of the natural childbirth movement has been the shift in emphasis back to the mother and her needs in hospital births. Practices that were once routine such as enemas and shaving pubic hair are no longer performed, and mothers are not confined to bed; in fact even epidurals allow some mobility. Midwives and hospital staff constantly review procedures and guidelines. They have accepted wholeheartedly the findings of much research from around the world that has proved the efficacy of mobility during labour.

An excellent study done in Latin America has shown that in a group of mothers having their first baby, the length of labour in those who were allowed to move around as they wanted to was only two-thirds that of the women who were confined to bed. When all mothers were considered, the mobile group were 25 per cent quicker in producing their babies than those who did not move around.

The study also found that 95 per cent of mothers who are left to themselves prefer to be upright and are more comfortable when upright. When mothers spend time in different positions in labour they report less pain and greater comfort when sitting, standing, kneeling or squatting.

The study concluded that in normal spontaneous labour, women who are allowed to assume a vertical position have an easier progress through labour, shorten its duration and have less discomfort and pain. In the light of all this, no doctor or midwife would now deny women who are having normal labours the right to choose the position or positions that they find most comfortable during the first and second stages of labour, since this is likely to be the most advantageous position for them in terms of their pelvic shape and the position of the baby. Lying on the back for delivery is now positively discouraged for the reasons given below.

POSITIONS FOR DELIVERY

Before the end of the seventeenth century when labour rooms were solely the province of women, no one considered that the normal behaviour of a woman in childbirth should be interfered with. She was allowed to move about as she wanted, take up any position that she felt was comfortable, eat and drink as she wished and assume her chosen position for delivering the baby. Then doctors invaded the delivery room and at that time all doctors were men. A doctor at the French royal court proposed that women should lie on their backs in preference to using upright positions and birthing stools to make vaginal examinations and obstetric manoeuvres easier, not because it might benefit the mother or the baby.

It is natural for a woman to take up a semi-vertical position for delivery of the baby, not just because it's comfortable but because it is mechanically most efficient. When she is upright the uterine contractions are aiming downwards, pushing the baby out towards the floor. When a woman pushes she strains downwards in the same direction and most importantly the force of gravity helps the birth too.

When a woman lies on her back, the uterine contractions push the baby into the bed and not down the birth canal so the added advantage of the force of gravity is lost. The result is that the recumbent woman has to push her baby up and against the force of gravity. This not only prolongs labour but makes it more likely that complications may occur (see below left).

In most units women are allowed to give birth in a position that they find comfortable. If a ventouse or forceps delivery is necessary your legs may be put in stirrups, so that the doctor is able to use the instruments most effectively and follow the contours of the pelvis while delivering the baby. This will mean less trauma for the mother.

However, even in these circumstances you will be propped up with pillows, not lying flat.

DISADVANTAGES OF LYING ON YOUR BACK FOR DELIVERY

If you lie on your back:
● your blood pressure may drop, thus reducing the amount of blood and oxygen to the baby
● pain is greater in this position than in a vertical one
● there is a greater need for an episiotomy
● there is an increased chance of a forceps delivery
● it inhibits spontaneous delivery of the placenta
● there is a greater possibility of low back strain in this position.

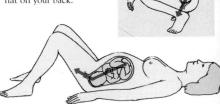

DELIVERY POSITION
It is more efficient to give birth in a semi-vertical position. The force of gravity helps to push the baby down and out rather than into the bed, which happens if you are lying flat on your back.

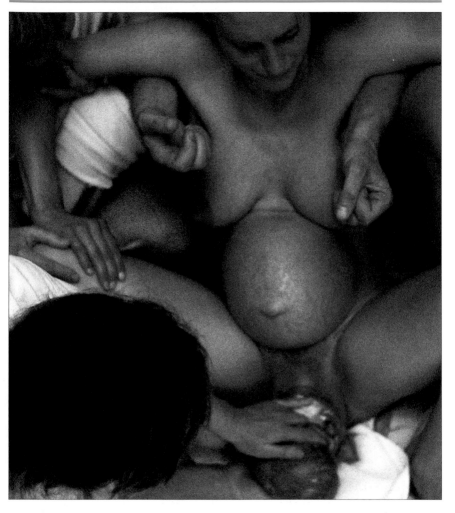

KEEPING UPRIGHT
More and more women now prefer to give birth in a vertical or semi-vertical position. The force of gravity helps to push the baby out.

FOOD AND DRINK

During labour the stomach seems to close down, and any food eaten during this time may be vomited up. For this reason it is a good idea to have something light and easily digestible to eat very early in labour while you are still at home to give you reserves of energy. Take glucose tablets into the delivery room with you in case you have a sudden demand for energy.

Most women can eat or drink during labour if they wish, but those at high risk of needing an emergency general anaesthetic will be advised not to.

However, I don't believe that this is a good enough reason to withhold food from all women – it should only be an option for those who are definitely at risk of needing a surgical procedure.

Most women in labour don't want to eat but most do require fluids, particularly as labour advances and fluids are lost through sweating, so water should be given, in my opinion, whenever it is requested. If a mother starts to become dehydrated during labour, an intravenous drip may have to be set up to administer glucose solution directly to the mother's bloodstream, bypassing the stomach and thereby increasing the medical intervention in her labour.

THE DELIVERY ROOM

In most hospitals nowadays you will go through your labour and deliver your baby in the same room. The only time you are likely to be moved is if you have to have an emergency Caesarean – most delivery rooms are not big enough to accommodate all the equipment safely.

At your antenatal clinic ask about the delivery rooms. Most hospital-based antenatal classes will include a tour of the delivery suite and postnatal wards; try to do this so you know what to expect.

Most delivery rooms now have soft lighting, pictures on the walls and pleasant, homely soft furnishings. There will be a bed (not an old-fashioned delivery table), but you may also be able to use a mat on the floor or a beanbag for back support. Some of the more progressive units make birthing pools available as an aid to pain relief. If there is no pool in the hospital you are going to, and there is an appropriate room and the staff are amenable, it may be possible for you to hire one.

You can also use aromatherapy during labour: to perfume the birthing pool, in massage oil and on your pillow. Ask what is available in your hospital and what you can bring with you to make your labour as comfortable as possible. You'll be able to deliver almost exactly as if you are at home but with medical facilities on tap should either you or your baby need them.

Choosing how to feed

THE MOST IMPORTANT ASPECT of infant feeding is feeding the infant. Most babies thrive whether they are breast or bottle fed. Given that as a basis (and in your worst moments remind yourself of this as your over-riding priority), think about the other considerations.

In order to make a choice and exercise an option you have to be aware of the pros and cons of breast and bottle feeding or a combination of both. You must bear in mind your own preferences because feeding will be most successful if you are happy with the method you have chosen. And you must also think about what is best for your baby. Although bottle feeding is convenient, there's little doubt that where the baby's well-being is concerned, breastfeeding is superior.

ADVANTAGES OF BREASTFEEDING

• A good reason for breastfeeding is that it's the natural thing to do. Most women have a natural urge to breastfeed, and there are very few women who are not physically equipped to breastfeed. No matter how small the breasts, they will be able to produce enough milk to feed and sustain the baby. Even women whose nipples are inverted can, with early diagnosis, breastfeed their babies (see p. 57).
• It's natural for a mother to feel proud that her baby is being fed on food that she provides and it's natural to crave the physical nearness and pleasure and to know that you are helping a close relationship to develop between you and your child.

• Breastfed babies are less liable to illness than bottle-fed ones. There are fewer cases of gastroenteritis, chest infection and measles. All the mother's antibodies to bacterial and viral infections are present in the colostrum, the first milk made by the breasts that is present in the breasts from the fifth month of pregnancy. In the first few days of life, therefore, when the baby is taking only the high-protein colostrum, she is living under the umbrella of her mother's antibodies. They have a protective effect in the intestine but also, as they're absorbed straight into the baby's system unchanged, they form an important part of the baby's own protection against infections. Take the example of a mother who has antibodies to poliomyelitis in her own body. Because those antibodies appear in her colostrum, it's not possible to infect her baby with the poliomyelitis virus while she's being wholly breastfed. The antibodies in the baby's gut will kill the virus before it can do any harm. Besides that, human milk is antibacterial because it contains substances that destroy bacteria. Even though these substances are present in cow's milk, a bottle-fed baby is not protected in the same way because the antibodies are inactivated when the cow's milk is heated.

• Human breast milk is the best source of food for a human baby; it has just the right amount of minerals and proteins. Cow's milk, which is for calves, has a higher percentage of protein and a high content of casein, which is the least digestible part of it and is passed out in the stool in the form of curds.

• Human milk contains just the right amount of sodium (salt) for a newborn baby. This is important because the immature kidneys of the infant are unable to deal with high levels of sodium in the blood. Cow's milk contains more sodium than human milk.

• While human milk and cow's milk contain the same amount of fat, the droplets in human milk are smaller and more digestible. Breast milk fat is high in polyunsaturates and low in cholesterol, and it may therefore protect against heart disease in later life. Breast milk also contains more sugar (lactose) than cow's milk and the mineral and vitamin content is different.

• Breastfeeding is good for the figure. Research has shown that a woman loses most of the fat she's accumulated during pregnancy if she breastfeeds. If you don't feed your baby yourself, you'll probably have more difficulty returning to your pre-pregnancy weight.

• It's a common fallacy that the breasts lose their shape and firmness through breastfeeding. This is not so. The changes that occur in the breasts are a consequence of becoming pregnant, not of producing milk or feeding your baby.

• Breastfeeding also has the advantage that it releases the hormone oxytocin which encourages the uterus to shrink to its non-pregnant size, hastening the return to normal of the pelvis and your waistline.

• The sheer convenience of breastfeeding also mustn't be ignored. Milk is always available for the baby at any time of the day or night, it doesn't have to be warmed up, there's no expensive equipment to buy and keep sterile, and it's free.

• Bonding occurs between mother and baby quite automatically if you breastfeed. When a baby is at the breast, her face is close to her mother's face – about 20–25cm (8–10in) – and even a newborn baby can focus at this distance (see p. 148). The act of making eye contact and smiling at your baby as she sucks, helps to create a physical and emotional bond between mother and baby which is hardly ever broken for the rest of their lives.

PROBLEMS OF BREASTFEEDING

One of the often quoted disadvantages of breastfeeding is that it curtails social activity. This need not necessarily be so. During the early weeks babies are very portable and you can take your baby with you when you go out. Although feeding in public places can still cause raised eyebrows, it's easy to feed discreetly, and many stores, restaurants, train terminals and airports now have designated baby-feeding areas.

• If you don't want to take your baby with you, you can take off sufficient milk with a breast pump to serve the baby's needs while you're away from her. You can bottle your own breast milk in sterile bottles and store them in the fridge or freezer and your babysitter can give the bottle to your baby later on your behalf. Remember, even if you only feed your

baby for two weeks, that's better than not breastfeeding at all and it will give your baby a flying start in life. Incidentally, one of the advantages of expressing some of your milk into bottles is that your partner can then become involved with the feeding routine too.

BOTTLE FEEDING

• As there are no real arguments against breastfeeding, it is also true to say that there are no arguments in favour of bottle

---

BREASTFEEDING AFTER A CAESAREAN

You may fear if you are advised to have a Caesarean delivery, that it will be too uncomfortable to breastfeed in the first weeks after the birth, so you may feel you should opt to bottle feed from the start. However, your midwife or obstetric physiotherapist will show you comfortable positions for breastfeeding so that the baby does not press against your wound. One way

is to lay your baby on pillows on your lap, or to tuck your baby's body under your arm with her head close to your breast. Alternatively you can lay your baby down next to you as shown below.

LYING DOWN TO BREASTFEED
You can lay your baby next to you while you lie down so she can feed from your lower breast. This is also a good way to breastfeed in bed at night.

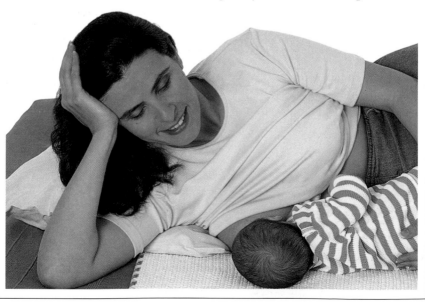

feeding. However, for you in your particular circumstances with your particular predilections, breastfeeding may not be a feasible or workable alternative, in which case bottle feeding will be your choice. If it is, don't feel that your child is getting second best.

● Babies thrive and are perfectly happy being bottle fed, and always remember that your baby needs your love and care more than she needs your breast milk. Bottle feeding, love and attention are an excellent option for any baby.

● There will be certain mothers who don't have any option but to bottle feed. These are women who may be taking drugs in the long term for a medical condition, such as epilepsy which needs barbiturates to keep it under control, or chronic depression for which antidepressants are prescribed. You may become seriously ill and need admission to hospital. If physically you're not in a fit state to breastfeed, then you should not. If you have to take any medicines regularly, discuss with your doctor whether they are passed on to your baby in breast milk and what the possible effects will be on breastfeeding and your baby. Quite often it's possible for nursing mothers to change to safer drugs.

● Some handicapped babies, or babies with physical abnormalities such as cleft palate or deformity of the jaw and mouth, may not be able to suck the breast successfully and will have to be spoon or bottle fed.

● If you think your milk supply is inadequate and the baby is failing to thrive, consult your midwife or a breastfeeding counsellor before opting to bottle feed. Your own nutrition and physical fitness do have a bearing on successful breastfeeding so you need to pay attention to getting a balanced diet (see p. 70).

● Some women have a strong physical revulsion against breastfeeding and find it a tiresome chore. A woman who feels revulsion very strongly will be under stress, and this may interfere both with milk production and milk flow. If you feel that your baby is not getting enough, these negative messages will also reinforce your dislike of breastfeeding. If this happens to you, do try to talk over your feelings before the birth of your baby with a sympathetic friend or midwife and do involve your baby's father.

● One of the main advantages of bottle feeding is that your partner can be equally involved in feeding your baby from the outset, which allows him to create a close, nurturing bond with his baby. It also means that you can work out a shared feeding schedule which gives you each enough time for rest, for unbroken sleep and time off for yourselves.

● One of the questionable advantages of bottle feeding is that babies sleep longer between feeds during the first weeks (although this is by no means always the case). This longer sleeping period could be because the casein content of cow's milk is higher than that of human milk and takes longer to digest.

● With bottle feeding, you can see exactly how much milk your baby has taken, which can be most reassuring.

PROBLEMS WITH BOTTLE FEEDING

● The posset from a bottle-fed baby has an unpleasant smell, as do the stools.

● Some babies are allergic to the alien protein in cow's milk. There are soya substitutes for babies with allergies; nursing mothers in families with a history of eczema or asthma are advised to breastfeed or use these substitutes.

● The sterilization of bottle-feeding equipment and the careful preparation of feeds are time-consuming compared to the accessibility of breast milk.

● Bottle-fed babies are more prone to gastric infections than breastfed babies, who receive some protection from their mothers' milk.

● The cost of formula milk, bottles, teats and sterilizing equipment is substantial, whereas breastfeeding is free and is always available.

3

Antenatal care

Antenatal care is the key to healthy mothers, happy pregnancies and thriving babies and its importance can't be over-emphasized. It's now accepted by most doctors that the one way in which we can improve the statistics on childbirth is through early and vigorous antenatal care. For most women, attendance at antenatal clinics, whether in the hospital or a local surgery, is smooth and happy. By talking to other mothers and to doctors and midwives, you can find out more about pregnancy and birth, which should help to reassure you and make you feel more confident about forthcoming events. Much of the antenatal care is routine, but at the clinic you can ask questions and explore the different circumstances in which you can have your baby so that you can plan ahead to get the kind of birth you want.

Going to the doctor

AS SOON AS YOU SUSPECT or know that you are pregnant, make an appointment to go to see your doctor. He or she will want to know the date of the first day of your last menstrual period (LMP) as it is from this day that the pregnancy is measured. Depending on how far your pregnancy is advanced, your doctor will perform some kind of pregnancy test – either a urine test (see p. 20) or a blood test if you have missed at least one menstrual period. He or she may want to confirm the pregnancy even if you have already used a home kit yourself and know that you're definitely pregnant.

The first visit to your doctor is important not just for confirmation of the pregnancy. It's at this first meeting that you can discuss in general terms the options for birth (see pp. 26–41), so give the subject some thought before you go along, for example whether you would like a home or hospital birth. Your preferences may conflict with your doctor's desire to stick to routines and procedures that he or she is used to and is reluctant to change, particularly with regard to home births. It's helpful for your partner to accompany you to this first appointment so you can discuss these issues together and iron out any difficulties from the start.

If you are over 35 or you have some history of genetic disorders in the family, your doctor may refer you for a chorionic biopsy (see p. 51). This procedure should be done around weeks 10–12, so visit your doctor early to get a letter of referral.

Use your doctor as a source of information: ask for a list of recommended books to read and pamphlets to send off for. If your own doctor does not specialize in obstetrics, he or she may pass you on to another member of the practice, or you may even be referred to a neighbouring practice where they undertake antenatal care and home confinement if this is what you want.

The other option is to attend the local hospital or the hospital of your choice depending on your area, in which case you will be looked after by the medical staff at the hospital and not by your own doctor.

Antenatal clinics

AFTER CONFIRMATION of the pregnancy your doctor will make arrangements for your antenatal care. This will depend upon the sort of birth you want. Most antenatal care is now undertaken at community antenatal clinics run by midwifes, not at hospitals, so long waits in hospital are no longer the norm. You should only need to go to the hospital clinic for your first visit when you need to have a scan, blood tests and so on; you will only have to go more than once if there is a specific reason for you to be examined by an obstetrician, such as high blood pressure, which may be a sign of pre-eclampsia (pregnancy-induced high blood pressure), or if you have an underlying medical condition such as diabetes.

ANTENATAL CLASSES
You can find out about antenatal classes at your antenatal clinic. Attending classes as a couple can be enjoyable as well as helpful; you'll meet other couples whose pregnancies are at the same stage as yours and can compare notes with them.

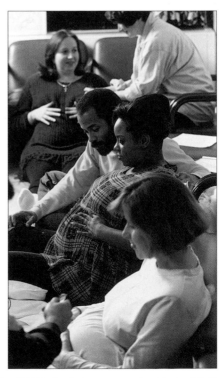

COPING AT THE CLINIC

These days, you shouldn't have to wait too long at the hospital antenatal clinic, but just in case try to make the best of your time there by preparing in the following ways:
● take along a friend to chat to or a good book or magazine to read
● take some water and a small snack such as some fruit with you in case it's difficult for you to get to the cafeteria
● make notes of all the questions you want to ask and note any worries even if you're not sure if they're linked to your pregnancy or not
● try to get your other children cared for while you go to the clinic; it's hard to keep them entertained so they may get bored and make you nervous.

ROUTINE ANTENATAL TESTS

NAME	PURPOSE	SIGNIFICANCE
HEIGHT 1st visit	To assess size of pelvis and pelvic outlet.	Very short height can suggest a small pelvic outlet and consequently maybe a difficult delivery.
WEIGHT occasionally	To check that weight gain or loss is not excessive.	Excessive weight gain may put undue strain on the heart. Sudden weight gain may indicate pre-eclampsia (pregnancy-induced high blood pressure).
BREASTS 1st visit only unless there is a problem	Check for lumps and condition of nipples. Breasts are not always examined, but if you are concerned about any aspect of your breast health, mention it to your midwife.	If nipples are retracted and you wish to breastfeed, you may be advised to wear a breast shield (see p. 57), do gentle exercises on the nipples or just wait and see. They may correct themselves during the pregnancy.
LUNGS, HAIR, EYES, TEETH, NAILS 1st visit	To check on your general physical health.	You may need some special attention and dietary supplements (see p. 75) or just general advice on diet. Dental visits will be encouraged.
LEGS AND HANDS every visit	To look for varicose veins and any swelling (oedema) in the ankles, hands or fingers.	Cases of extreme puffiness can be a sign of pre-eclampsia (pregnancy-induced high blood pressure). Advice on what to do about varicose veins will be given.
URINE (MSU) 1st visit	To test for kidney infection. After cleaning the vulva with sterile pads, you pass a sample of urine into a sterile container. Allow the first drops to go into the toilet bowl and collect the mid-stream urine (MSU) only.	An existing kidney infection you may not know you have can develop into a serious condition in pregnancy. You will be treated with antibiotics.
URINE every visit	1 Tests for protein in case your kidneys aren't coping well. 2 Tests for the presence of sugar; if sugar is found repeatedly, you may have diabetes. 3 Tests for ketones.	1 Protein in urine late in pregnancy is a sign of pre-eclampsia (pregnancy-induced high blood pressure). Bed rest will probably be prescribed. 2 Pregnancy can unmask diabetes, which must be treated and stabilized. It may go away after delivery only to return in later pregnancies. 3 Presence of ketones indicates that the body is short of sugar. This may be a sign of diabetes – if so, further tests will be made to confirm it and you will be treated accordingly. Alternatively you may simply not be eating enough and you'll be given advice on an adequate diet.
FETAL HEART- BEAT after week 14	To confirm that the fetus is alive and that the heart and heart rate are normal.	If the midwife listens to your baby's heart with a sonicaid (this listens to the fetal heart with ultrasound vibrations), the sound of the beat will be amplified and you will be able to hear it too.

NAME	PURPOSE	SIGNIFICANCE
ABDOMINAL PALPATION every visit after 24 weeks	To assess the height of the fundus (the top of the uterus – see p. 59), and the size and position of the fetus.	Gives a guide to the length of the pregnancy and the lie of the fetus in the womb. Palpation after 36 weeks indicates the lie of the fetus. This may indicate whether the baby is in the breech position (see p. 144).
BLOOD PRESSURE every visit	This is the measurement of the pressure at which the heart is pumping blood through your body. The test is done to assess if it is normal or not. The reading is made up of two numbers: the top one is the systolic pressure, when the heart contracts, pushes out blood and "beats". This can be heard when the arm band is tightened; the bottom one is the diastolic pressure, the resting pressure between heartbeats. A normal BP is 120/70.	Hypertension (high blood pressure) can indicate a number of problems, including pre-eclampsia (pregnancy-induced high blood pressure that suddenly rises, e.g. above 140/90). Constant checks mean it can be kept under control. May mean bed rest in hospital if it rises. Any rise in the lower or diastolic figure is cause for concern.
BLOOD TESTS 1st visit: tests 1, 2, 3, 5, 6, 7, 8 16 weeks; test 4 28 weeks: tests 1, 2, 3	1 To find your major blood group: A, B, or O. 2 To find your Rhesus blood group. 3 To find your haemoglobin level (repeated test). This is a measure of the oxygen-carrying substances in your red blood cells. Normal levels, measured in gm., are between 12 and 14gm. 4 Alpha-fetoprotein levels – a special test at 16 weeks (see p. 49). 5 To detect the presence of German measles antibodies. 6 VDRL, Kahn or Wasserman tests for the presence of syphilis. 7 To detect or confirm sickle cell disease and thalassaemia, both forms of anaemia mainly found in dark-skinned people and those from the Mediterranean region. 8 To check whether the mother is HIV positive (done by consent).	1 Blood group needed in case of an emergency transfusion. 2 In case of Rhesus incompatibility. 3 During pregnancy your haemoglobin level may drop, because pregnant women have more circulating blood (see p. 60), but if it goes below 10gm, treatment for anaemia will be given. Iron and folic acid supplements will raise the haemoglobin level so that more oxygen can be carried to the baby. 4 See p. 49. 5 To find out whether or not you have immunity to rubella; if not you will be warned not to come into contact with German measles during your pregnancy. 6 If you unknowingly have this sexually transmitted infection, it is essential to treat it before week 20 of your pregnancy; after this time it can be passed to the baby. 7 Both of these conditions can affect the baby and the pregnancy. If either condition is found and youwere not already aware of it, you will be given folic acid supplements. 8 Antibodies can cross the placenta to the baby. The baby will probably be delivered by Caesarean.

THE FIRST VISIT

The purpose of your first visit to the antenatal clinic at around 12 weeks is to give information to the staff so that they can judge whether or not your pregnancy and delivery will be normal. If you want to have a home delivery, you will be asked about the social and domestic side of your life to assess whether your circumstances are suitable for home delivery.

The staff will also run certain tests on you to see if you are healthy (see p. 44); for instance, taking your blood pressure, collecting a sample of your blood and testing your urine. Blood and urine tests

YOUR ANTENATAL FILE

At the initial interview you will be asked some or all of the following questions about your relevant medical and past obstetric history:
● your name, age, race, date and place of birth, and your date of marriage, if any, and the name of your next of kin
● about your childhood illnesses, and whether or not you have ever been in hospital or had any serious disease or any surgical operations
● if any illnesses run in your family or your partner's family
● whether there are twins in either family
● whether you used contraceptives, if so what sort and when you stopped
● about your menstrual history: when your periods first started, how long your average cycle is, how many days you bleed and the date of the first day of your last menstrual period
● whether you have any pregnancy symptoms and what your general state of health is like
● about the births of any other children you may have, or any miscarriages
● whether you are taking any prescription medicines or suffer from any allergies
● what work you and your partner do and whether you are still working.

THE CLINIC

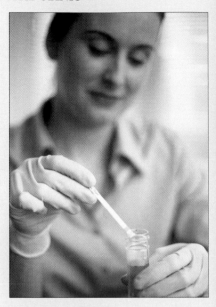

TESTING YOUR URINE
At every antenatal visit you will be asked to supply a sample of your urine. Routine tests will be done immediately and the results marked in your notes.

may have to be sent away to a laboratory and the results will come back later and be available at your next visit.

Ask questions, too. It's important for you to gain confidence in your pregnancy by expressing any concerns. It isn't essential now at the first visit, but it's as well to discuss your preferences for pain relief during the labour, whether you want an early discharge, and what course of action you want if the baby is overdue. Your file and notes will be made available to you.

At the end of the visit you may be given iron tablets (see p. 75) and you can ask to see a dietitian if you need information about diet and nutrition. You will probably attend the antenatal clinic

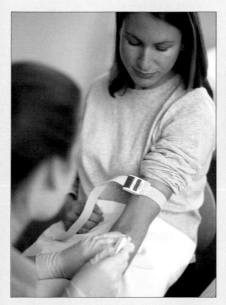

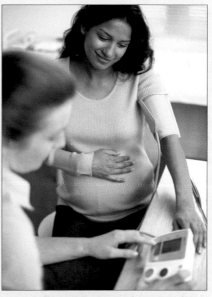

TAKING A BLOOD SAMPLE
A routine sample of your blood will be taken twice during pregnancy, and tested for specific problems and as a general check on your health. The blood sample taken at your first antenatal appointment is sometimes also used to confirm the pregnancy.

TAKING YOUR BLOOD PRESSURE
This is measured at every visit so that any change can be quickly brought under control. Raised blood pressure may be a sign of pre-eclampsia, so you will be closely monitored by your doctor and midwife.

every four to six weeks up to 36 weeks, and thereafter every two to three weeks. Check-ups are more flexible than they used to be, and their frequency will depend on your health and the health of your baby.

When you enrol at an antenatal clinic you'll be told about the antenatal classes and will be given details of where they're held and at what time.

THE MEDICAL STAFF

● The midwife is a nurse with special training in the care of normal pregnant women and the delivery of their babies. If all goes well a midwife will deliver your baby whether at home or in hospital.

Midwives also work in the community and once you return home after delivery, you will be visited by a midwife every day until 10 days after the birth.
● Your family doctor may be responsible for part of your antenatal care. He or she may attend your delivery at home, although family doctors do not routinely attend home births; if all is well they are happy to leave it to the midwife.
● The obstetrician is the hospital doctor who specializes in pregnancy and birth, and he or she heads the team of midwives, nurses and other doctors who provide your antenatal care and deliver your baby. The consultant obstetrician usually attends only the difficult births.

UNDERSTANDING YOUR HOSPITAL NOTES

At your first antenatal visit you will be given your hospital notes. At every visit your doctor or midwife will record on them details of the routine tests and the progress of the pregnancy. Take your notes with you to every clinic. Keep them with you if you go out of your area – if you should need medical attention, all the information will be at hand. Most of the abbreviations are explained below.

NAD/nil/✓	Nothing abnormal discovered in urine
Alb	Albumin in urine (a name for one of the proteins found in urine)
BP	Blood pressure
FHH/NH	Fetal heart heard or not heard
FH	Fetal heart
FMF	Fetal movements felt
Ceph.	Cephalic, the baby is head down
Vx	Vertex, the baby is head down
Br.	Breech, the baby is bottom down
LMP	Last menstrual period
EDD/EDC	Estimated date of delivery or confinement
Hb	Haemoglobin levels to check for anaemia
Eng/E	Engaged, the baby's head has dropped into the pelvis ready for birth
NE	Not engaged
Para O	Woman has no other children
Para 1 (etc)	Woman has one child
Fe	Iron has been prescribed
TCA	To come again
PET	Pre-eclamptic toxaemia
Long L	Longitudinal lie, the baby is parallel to your spine in the womb

Height of fundus	The height of the top of the uterus. The baby pushes this up as it grows and often the height is used to estimate the length of the pregnancy. Some clinics measure the height of the fundus (from the top of the pubic bone to the top of the uterus) with a tape measure in centimetres. This figure is usually roughly the same as the pregnancy in weeks.
Relation of PP to brim	This is the brim of your pelvis. The presenting part (PP) of the baby to the brim in the later stages of your pregnancy will be the part in your cervix ready to be born first.
Oed.	Oedema
RSA	Right sacrum anterior – the most common breech position
AFP	Alpha fetoprotein
CS	Caesarean section
H/T	Hypertension
MSU	Mid-stream urine sample
Primigravida	First pregnancy
Multigravida	More than one pregnancy
VE	Vaginal examination

THE LIE OF THE BABY
Certain abbreviations describe the way the baby is lying in the womb (see pp. 117 and 144). They refer to the position of the crown of the baby's head (occiput) in relation to your body; that is whether on the right or the left, to the front (anterior) or back (posterior).

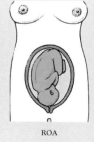

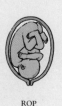

ROA   LOA   ROP   LOP

THE OLDER WOMAN

Nowadays the age of the mother is much less important than her medical history, diet and lifestyle. However, if you're over 35, you may still be asked extra questions at your first antenatal appointment. Once all the questions have been answered, any tests performed (see below), and you're found to be generally fit and well, your care will be no different from that of younger women.

PARENTCRAFT CLASSES

First-time parents can gain confidence and information from these classes. They should ideally cover an understanding of pregnancy and birth; techniques of relaxation and breathing to prepare for labour; and caring for a small baby. Hospital-run classes will help you understand the procedures in that hospital and you will be able to see the delivery suite and postnatal wards.

Special tests

THERE ARE A NUMBER of tests available to check for any potential physical or chromosomal abnormality in the fetus. The tests include alpha fetoprotein (AFP) screening or the triple test, and invasive techniques such as amniocentesis or chorionic villus sampling (CVS). None of the tests detailed here is compulsory and a few, such as the triple test, are only available at specialist centres. Discuss them with your midwife or doctor.

AFP SCREENING

Alpha fetoprotein (AFP) is a substance found in the blood of a pregnant woman that varies in level throughout the pregnancy. Between 16 and 18 weeks the levels are usually low, so if your blood is examined for AFP at this time, and the levels are raised, you could be carrying a baby with a neural tube defect such as spina bifida, or other abnormalities of brain development. The test is no longer used to assess the risk of Down's syndrome, which is now checked for by a nuchal translucency scan (see p. 51).

Raised AFP levels in the blood are not, however, conclusive evidence of neural tube defect. In addition, AFP levels may be raised with a twin pregnancy and may also rise as pregnancy progresses. If a blood test indicates raised levels, an ultrasound scan will be taken to check for twins or to confirm your dates in case the pregnancy is more advanced than you thought. A further blood test will then be taken. Only if these checks prove positive and if corroboration is needed will amniocentesis be contemplated because to be certain, alpha fetoprotein must also be found in abnormal quantities in the amniotic fluid. Minor neural tube defects such as a small hairy mole at the bottom of the spine are quite common.

Lower than normal levels of AFP indicate the risk of Down's syndrome; in this case amniocentesis will be offered.

TRIPLE TEST

The triple test is another maternal serum screening test, also known as the Bart's triple test, the Leeds test, the Biomark, or the Beta Triple. An extension of the AFP test, it also measures other hormones present in the woman's blood, such as oestriol and human chorionic gonadotrophin. The test is done in the 16th week of pregnancy, and the results take about two weeks to come through. The results can be assessed alongside your age to predict the chance of your baby suffering from Down's syndrome. If the chances seem high, amniocentesis will be offered. The triple test is not offered in all centres, although you can request it, and you may have to pay for it.

ULTRASOUND

This works by giving a photographic picture that is formed by creating images from the echoes of sound waves bouncing off different parts of the body of different consistencies. Unlike X-rays, ultrasound can show soft tissue in detail and will give a very accurate picture of the fetus in the uterus. Ultrasound is very useful as a way of determining the age of the fetus, the position of the placenta and therefore your expected date of delivery. Any visible abnormalities will be picked up clearly by the scan technician.

The first scan is often given at around 11–13 weeks of pregnancy, to establish the age of the fetus, and for nuchal translucency (see p. 51). A second scan given at 20–22 weeks will check that your baby is growing properly. The scan can take 20 minutes or more.

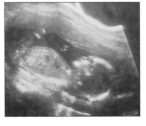

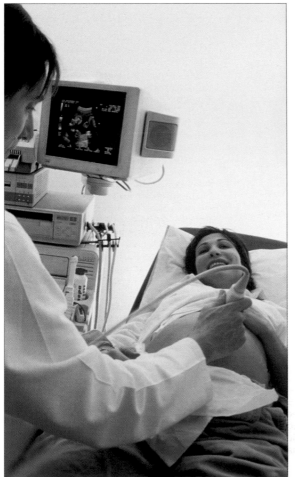

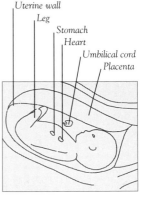

Uterine wall
Leg
Stomach
Heart
Umbilical cord
Placenta

THE FETUS IN UTERO

It is very exciting to see a picture of your baby moving about in your womb. The shapes may not make much sense to you so ask the technician to point out the head, limbs and the baby's organs. The ultrasound procedure is painless but if you have a scan in the early part of your pregnancy you will need to have a full bladder. Don't worry about this; arrive early and drink several glasses of water.

You will have been asked beforehand not to pass urine and, if it is an early scan, to drink plenty of fluids so that your bladder is full and clearly visible to the technician. Wear loose clothes so you can easily lift them off your abdomen. Warm oil or jelly is spread onto your stomach and a transducer is passed over it, which sends back signals onto a black and white monitor. You will feel no pain at all, just a soft, oily, flowing sensation.

USES OF ULTRASOUND

An ultrasound scan is used by medical staff to:
● help determine the age of the fetus by taking measurements of the head and body. If the scan is done early in pregnancy, it will be accurate to within one week
● measure growth, and growth retardation when clinical examination suggests something is wrong. Serial assessment – that is, a number of scans over a period of time – monitors fetal growth and establishes the estimated date of delivery
● find out the exact position of the baby and placenta before an amniocentesis (see p. 52)
● locate the position of the placenta and its condition, should it become dislodged late in pregnancy
● determine if you are carrying more than one baby should alpha-fetoprotein levels start to rise
● pick up visible abnormalities of the baby such as brain or kidney conditions
● identify any growths in the mother that might hinder delivery.

NUCHAL TRANSLUCENCY SCAN

This is a special test used to assess the risk of Down's syndrome. A high-definition ultrasound scan can be carried out to measure the collection of fluid at the back of a baby's neck. All babies have some fluid, but a higher than normal reading can be an indication of an increased risk

of Down's syndrome. A high reading does not necessarily mean there is a problem, but it would indicate the need for further tests, such as chorionic villus sampling or amniocentesis, to be done. The NT test should be carried out between weeks 11 and 13 of your pregnancy, and research studies have shown it to be about 75 per cent accurate. When combined with a blood test the accuracy rate rises to about 90 per cent.

CHORIONIC VILLUS SAMPLING

If you have a family history of genetic disorders, such as sickle cell anaemia, haemophilia or cystic fibrosis, or if you have had an affected baby previously, it is likely you will see the obstetrician early in pregnancy. This gives you a chance to discuss prenatal testing such as chorionic villus sampling (CVS), which is usually done at 10 to 12 weeks.

The CVS test takes about 10–20 minutes. A small sample of the chorion (the outer tissue that surrounds the developing fetus and placenta) is taken and analysed. Using an ultrasound scan to guide the probe, a fine hollow tube is inserted in the vagina or through the abdominal wall and into the uterus. A few of the chorionic cells are sucked out; these cells are identical to those in the fetus. The chromosomal analysis of the cells taken from the chorion gives a "window" onto the fetus.

Very occasionally, CVS may lead to rupture of the amniotic sac, infection and bleeding. Even so, it only seems to increase the risk of miscarriage by one per cent.

This test is performed earlier in pregnancy than amniocentesis and the results are available in about 10 days. CVS therefore gives the woman the choice of an early termination, rather than having to wait 15–18 weeks for an amniocentesis and then waiting a further three weeks for the results. If you think the test might be helpful, discuss it with your doctor or midwife early in pregnancy, as well as with your partner or a friend.

AMNIOCENTESIS

Used to detect a range of chromosomal defects, amniocentesis is not a routine test and is carried out only if certain hereditary or sex-linked disorders run in your family, or if the obstetrician suspects some abnormality that cannot be detected by other tests. Though it is readily available, it is still a serious interference with your pregnancy. It involves taking a sample of the fluid surrounding the baby in the uterus. Any discarded cells floating in the amniotic fluid will give an accurate chromosome count and denote abnormal chromosomal structure. It is also possible to find out how much oxygen and carbon dioxide is in the fluid, revealing whether the baby is getting sufficient oxygen.

Many women over 35 are concerned to see if their baby has any abnormalities. If you are worried, talk to your obstetrician. Most obstetricians will agree to this test to give you peace of mind. They will also recommend amniocentesis if you already have an abnormal child, or if there is a family history of abnormality. The sex of the baby can be determined by simply looking at some cells of the skin so you can find out if any gender-linked disorders might have been inherited. However, doctors will not do the test simply to find out the baby's sex. In cases of Rhesus incompatibility, the bilirubin content of the fluid is a good indicator as to whether the baby needs an intrauterine blood transfusion.

HOW AMNIOCENTESIS WORKS

Amniotic fluid is swallowed by the fetus and passed out through its mouth or bladder; this fluid contains cells from the skin and other organs that provide clues under analysis to the baby's condition. Amniocentesis is the procedure to extract this fluid from the womb. About 75 different genetic diseases can then be subjected to chromosome analysis. The test is done in hospital, generally not until 14–16 weeks after the last menstrual period; before then there is unlikely to be sufficient fluid in the amniotic sac and therefore not enough cells to analyse.

HAVING AN AMNIOCENTESIS
Amniotic fluid is drawn off from the womb and then analysed to determine the health of the baby.

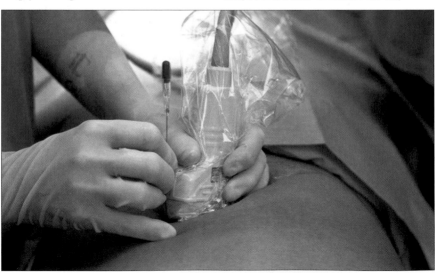

RISKS OF AMNIOCENTESIS

With a skilled operator and the use of an ultrasonic scan to show the exact position of the placenta and the fetus, the risk of miscarriage is less than that with CVS (see p. 51) – below one per cent in Britain, 0.5 per cent in the United States. When deciding to have amniocentesis you need to weigh up the reasons for you being offered it against the risk of miscarriage, and think about whether you are prepared to have your pregnancy terminated if the results give cause for concern.

Possibly the worst element of amniocentesis is the stress of waiting for the result, although this should be no more than three weeks. Also your amniotic fluid may only be tested for a single abnormality, which means that a negative result may not reflect other possible problems. Ask your doctor for the results of all possible tests that could apply to you.

HOW THE FLUID IS EXTRACTED

After an ultrasonic scan to determine the position of the fetus and the placenta, a small area of the abdomen is numbed with local anaesthetic and a long hollow needle surmounted by a syringe is carefully inserted into the womb. About 14g (½ oz) of fluid is then drawn out.

The cells shed by the baby are then separated from the amniotic liquid in a centrifuge.

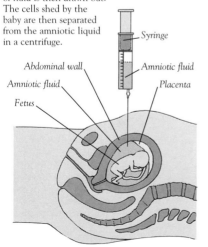

Syringe

Abdominal wall
Amniotic fluid
Amniotic fluid
Placenta
Fetus

REASONS FOR AMNIOCENTESIS

● Amniocentesis will be offered if you are over 35, when the risk of chromosomal abnormalities increases greatly and you may be at risk of carrying a Down's syndrome baby, for example (see below).

● It will also be offered if you are a carrier of genetically linked disorders such as haemophilia, cystic fibrosis or certain forms of muscular dystrophy, where a male child will have a 50 per cent chance of being affected.

● The test can give parents the chance to decide whether they want to continue with the pregnancy. It also sometimes allows for early treatment of a disorder while the fetus is in the womb.

DOWN'S SYNDROME

This is the result of a chromosomal abnormality in the baby. In most cases an extra chromosome occurring before or immediately after fertilization gives the fetus 47 chromosomes in each cell instead of the normal 46. The exact cause is unknown but maternal age is an important factor, the risk of having a Down's syndrome baby rising sharply after the age of 35.

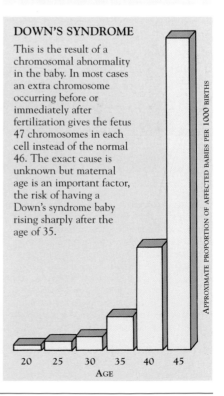

APPROXIMATE PROPORTION OF AFFECTED BABIES PER 1000 BIRTHS

20 25 30 35 40 45
AGE

4

Physical changes

Nearly all the changes in your body that you can see and feel, such as enlargement of the breasts, deepening pigmentation of the skin, and slight breathlessness on exertion, are due in one way or another to the increased production of a range of pregnancy hormones. Early in pregnancy your ovaries are responsible for the main output, but very quickly the maternal supply begins to be overtaken by that from the placenta. The output of hormones is colossal. For instance, during the menstrual cycle, the maximum daily output of one key hormone, progesterone, would be a few milligrams a day, but towards the end of pregnancy this rises to as much as 250 mg a day. While progesterone output increases 50–60 times, that of another key hormone, oestrogen, increases 20–30 times. These hormones cause changes in your whole body's structure and processes so that it can support and nourish your developing baby throughout pregnancy.

The menstrual cycle

THE FIRST DEVIATION from normal hormonal patterns occurs very early in pregnancy. The menstrual cycle begins when a hormone (follicle-stimulating hormone – FSH) from the pituitary gland stimulates the development of an egg (ovum) in a follicle inside one of the ovaries. In a 28-day menstrual cycle, ovulation occurs around day 14 when the follicle bursts, discharging the ovum which starts to move down the Fallopian tube towards the uterus. It is helped by "fingers" at the end of the Fallopian tube which direct it on its way. At the same time, the lining of the uterus (endometrium) begins to thicken and

the mucus at the neck of the uterus (cervix) becomes thinner so that the sperm can gain an easier entry. If the ovum is not fertilized, at around day 24 the decaying follicle (corpus luteum) begins to wither, and further hormonal changes result in shedding of the endometrium and bleeding on day 28 and day 1 of the next cycle.

When pregnancy occurs, fertilization happens around day 14 of the cycle, then implantation of the fertilized ovum in the uterine wall begins some seven days after that, around day 21. There are three or four days between implantation and the usual regression of the corpus luteum. The body has only this short interval in which to stop the regression and suppress menstruation. This is probably achieved by a powerful hormone called human chorionic gonadotrophin (HCG), which is produced by the fertilized ovum and whose immediate function is thought to be the maintenance of a healthy corpus luteum and the levels of oestrogen and progesterone coming from the ovaries. In this way, the mother's body and the developing embryo, which at this stage is only a minute ball of cells, cooperate to keep the pregnancy intact.

The hormone levels of some pregnant women are not sufficiently increased to prevent some bleeding at the time of their first missed period. Slight breakthrough bleeding may occur at the time when the second and even third missed periods would have been due. The bleeding does not harm the baby. However, if hormonal levels are too low, a miscarriage will almost certainly occur.

THE PLACENTA

At implantation, part of the fertilized ovum puts out microscopic protrusions (chorionic villi) which embed themselves in the uterine wall. These villi become the placenta, which supplies food and oxygen to the baby and carries waste from it. During the first trimester, the placenta develops into an efficient chemical factory, producing an ever-increasing supply of pregnancy hormones that alter the mother's body to maintain the pregnancy and prepare for lactation, and also maintain healthy reproductive organs and the efficient function of the placenta, so keeping the baby well nourished.

28-DAY MENSTRUAL CYCLE

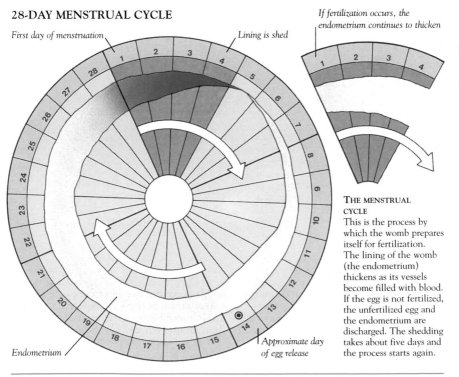

First day of menstruation

Lining is shed

If fertilization occurs, the endometrium continues to thicken

Endometrium

Approximate day of egg release

THE MENSTRUAL CYCLE

This is the process by which the womb prepares itself for fertilization. The lining of the womb (the endometrium) thickens as its vessels become filled with blood. If the egg is not fertilized, the unfertilized egg and the endometrium are discharged. The shedding takes about five days and the process starts again.

HORMONES OF PREGNANCY

NAME	ACTION	EFFECT ON MOTHER & BABY
HUMAN CHORIONIC GONADOTROPHIN (HCG)	Produced by the chorionic villi. Causes the ovary to produce more progesterone (see below), thus suppressing menstruation and sustaining the pregnancy. Reaches a peak of production around the 70th day and then falls to a constant value for the rest of the pregnancy. Maintains the function of the ovaries until the placenta takes over.	High levels in the bloodstream parallel the time when women normally suffer from nausea in pregnancy (see p. 19). Could be associated with morning sickness. Detection of this hormone in urine is a reliable pregnancy test (see p. 20).
HUMAN PLACENTAL LACTOGEN (HPL)	Produced by the placenta, it is essential to normal milk production.	Enlarges the breasts and causes secretion of colostrum from about the fifth month.
RELAXIN	Probably produced by the placenta. In animal experiments, it was found to soften the uterine cervix. Relaxes the pelvic joints.	May have an effect of relaxing the ligaments and joints.
OESTROGEN	Produced in the placenta using starter substances from the mother's and the baby's adrenal glands.	Affects all aspects of pregnancy. It is particularly important in maintaining the health of the genital tract, the reproductive organs and the breasts.
PROGESTERONE	Produced in the same way as oestrogen. Sustains the pregnancy, relaxes smooth muscle.	Affects all aspects of pregnancy. Prepares the breasts for lactation. Relaxation of joints and ligaments in preparation for childbirth can affect bowel movements, causing constipation, and can result in back pain. Raises body temperature.
MELANOCYTE STIMULATING HORMONE (MSH)	Produced in higher levels than normal during pregnancy. Stimulates the skin to produce pigment.	Increase in colour of the nipples, patches of brown pigmentation on the face, inner thighs and a brown line running down the centre of the abdomen (see p. 62). Some women notice none of these changes.

Breasts

SIZE AND SHAPE VARY from individual to individual and according to the point in the menstrual cycle. In the second half of the cycle, after ovulation day, most women experience some enlargement of their breasts. Just before menstruation, the consistency becomes rather nodular as the milk glands enlarge, the tinted areas around the nipples (areolas) become slightly bumpy as the sebaceous glands enlarge, and the nipples become sensitive. Changes in the breasts may be one of the earliest signs of pregnancy that you become aware of. Most women with an average 28-day cycle will notice a definite enlargement of the breasts by week 6–8 of

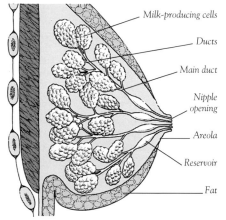

Milk-producing cells

Ducts

Main duct

Nipple opening

Areola

Reservoir

Fat

CROSS-SECTION OF THE BREAST
The breast is prepared for lactation during pregnancy by the action of oestrogen and progesterone.

pregnancy, two to four weeks after their first missed period would have started. The breasts will feel firm and generally tender and have more and larger veins than usual running close to the surface of the skin. Tingling is common, as are occasional stabbing pains. The sebaceous glands on the areolas (Montgomery's tubercles) become raised, nodular and pink.

The breasts are composed mainly of millions of tiny milk glands, plus their small ducts, that join to come out at the nipple. Although there is almost certainly some overlap in the effect of hormones, oestrogen stimulates the growth of the ducts while progesterone stimulates enlargement of the glands themselves. From early pregnancy your breasts will be making a form of milk called colostrum. This may be secreted involuntarily; it's nothing to worry about. If you find yourself leaking colostrum you may want to wear breast pads.

Most of the growth of the ducts and increase in size and weight of the breasts occurs in the first trimester. It is at this point that you should be fitted for a good bra. You will probably need one at least two sizes larger. You will also need feeding bras after the baby is born (see p. 97).

These should be fitted around a month before the baby is due. If you support the weight of your breasts during pregnancy and lactation they should return to their pre-pregnant shape and firmness when you stop breastfeeding. Some women find their breasts are smaller after weaning as the original fat in the breasts has been replaced by milk-producing ducts. Towards the end of the first trimester you will see one of the last changes in the breasts, darkening of the nipples and areolas due to a general increase in pigmentation (see p. 62) which is another characteristic of pregnancy.

INVERTED NIPPLES

If your nipples do not protrude when you are cold, sexually excited or breastfeeding, they are said to be flat or inverted. You can improve inverted nipples by wearing breast shields under your bra or you can try an exercise known as the Hoffmann technique. Place an index finger either side of the areola and stretch the nipples. Repeat this with your fingers placed above and below the areola. Do this a couple of times a day during pregnancy. Once you start breastfeeding the baby may help to solve the problem but could have difficulty latching on.

FLAT OR INVERTED NIPPLES
You can improve them by wearing breast shields under your bra from about week 15. Wear them for a few hours at first, building up to several hours each day in the third trimester. Made of plastic or glass, they have a hole in them through which the nipple is gently pulled by suction. It is not painful.

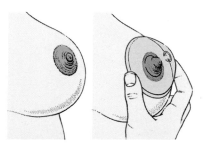

The uterus

THREE PRINCIPAL TASKS are performed by the uterus during pregnancy. It is the site of implantation by the fertilized ovum, it accommodates the growing baby, and it expels the baby at term. To achieve the second of these tasks the uterus has to grow and distend, while restraining a normal tendency to contract when there is something inside it and while the outlet, the cervix, remains resistant to stretching.

EXPANSION

To accommodate the developing baby, placenta and surrounding fluids, the internal volume of the uterus has to expand from being a potential space to one of about 5 litres (9 pints) – an increase in volume of some 1000 times. In the first half of pregnancy, the uterus gains weight quickly, mainly due to an increase in the size of the muscle fibres. Each muscle cell of the uterus increases in size by as much as 50 times, initially under the stimulation of oestrogen. Around mid-pregnancy this rate of growth slows down, but uterine volume then increases rapidly. The uterus increases its weight some 20 times, from about 40 g (1 ½ oz) to 800 g (28 oz) at term. The expansion is not noticeable until about week 16 when the uterus begins to rise out of the pelvis. By week 36 the top of the uterus has risen to just below the breast bone. When the baby's head engages (see p. 115), it descends again.

THE EXPANDING UTERUS
The uterus increases its volume about 1000 times in pregnancy and as it does, it crowds out the other organs. This can result in problems such as frequent urination, heartburn, breathlessness and constipation.

Diaphragm

Stomach

Intestines

Uterus

Fetus

Bladder

Vagina

Rectum

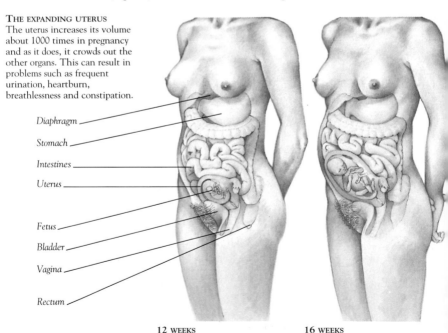

12 WEEKS
The uterus can just be felt by abdominal palpitation as it emerges out of the pelvic cavity.

16 WEEKS
The uterus is expanding quickly, your waist disappears and you are noticeably pregnant.

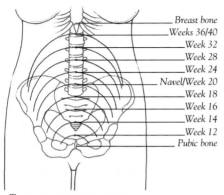

- Breast bone
- Weeks 36/40
- Week 32
- Week 28
- Week 24
- Navel/Week 20
- Week 18
- Week 16
- Week 14
- Week 12
- Pubic bone

THE HEIGHT OF THE FUNDUS
This can be determined by abdominal palpitation (feeling the abdomen) or by measuring in centimetres from the pubic bone. It is sometimes used as a guide to the duration of your pregnancy and is written on your notes.

CONTRACTIONS

One of the normal characteristics of uterine muscle is that it undergoes contractions which are hardly ever felt. All the way through pregnancy the uterus contracts in a weak, short-lived way that you may or may not notice, although if you put a hand on your abdomen you can feel the muscle going tight and hard. These slight, painless movements are called Braxton Hicks contractions and occur about every 20 minutes throughout pregnancy. They are important as they ensure a good blood circulation through the uterus and they help uterine growth. You probably won't notice Braxton Hicks contractions until the last month of your pregnancy. They can become quite strong and may be mistaken for labour. This is called "false labour" (see p. 117).

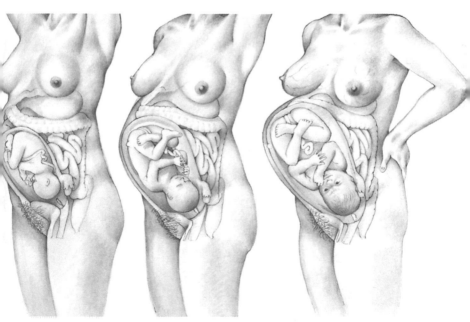

28 WEEKS
The skin on your stomach will start to stretch and the upward pressure may lead to indigestion.

36 WEEKS
The uterus is now putting pressure on your ribcage and you may feel a jabbing pain there.

40 WEEKS
The baby's head will engage in the pelvic cavity and put pressure on the groin and the pelvis.

Up until weeks 12–14, the developing baby can quite easily be accommodated in the space within the growing uterus, but after this time the junction of the uterus and the top of the cervix begins to smooth out, giving the baby more space. This part is called the lower segment of the uterus. While the upper half of the cervix is muscular and stretchy, the lower half contains a strong, tight band of fibrous tissue. This helps to prevent the cervix from dilating before the baby is ready to be born.

Although this band of fibrous tissue softens during the last weeks of pregnancy to prepare for the birth, its resistance to dilatation is usually sufficient to withstand Braxton Hicks contractions. During labour, it is the upper segment of the uterus that contracts to push the baby out.

Vagina

EARLY IN PREGNANCY, the vaginal tissues also change so that the vagina will dilate more easily for the birth. The muscle cells enlarge and the mucous membranes of the lining thicken. One side effect of this is an increase in vaginal secretions, which may mean you need light sanitary pads for comfort.

If the secretion has an offensive smell or makes you sore, tell your doctor and never douche during pregnancy. One other result of this increased lubrication and swelling of the vagina may be an increase in sexual pleasure. This, however, differs from woman to woman and will vary throughout the pregnancy (see p. 68).

Vital functions

YOUR BODY WILL REACT to the hormonal stimulation of pregnancy with widespread changes in the important circulatory, respiratory and urinary systems. It used to be thought that the relationship between the mother and embryo was simply that of host and parasite but we now know that it is much more complex. From the earliest days, in response to the diversified and raised hormonal output, the mother continually anticipates the needs of her baby: by changes in her vital functions, she precedes the baby's demands.

BLOOD

An average-sized, non-pregnant woman has about 5 litres (9 pints) of circulating blood. During pregnancy, the volume of blood increases by about 1.5 litres (2½ pints). The volume gradually increases from about week 10, reaching a plateau in the third trimester. The extra blood is required by the uterus (which takes about 25 per cent), the breasts and other vital organs – even the gums receive an increase in their blood supply (see p. 63). The increase in the liquid part of the blood (plasma) is proportionately greater than that of the red cells. If the red cells become too diluted, this will show up in antenatal blood tests as a fall in the haemoglobin concentration and this is known as physiological anaemia. It is not the same thing as iron-deficiency anaemia. In a normal pregnant woman, the number of red blood cells multiplies steadily, particularly if you include a lot of iron in your diet.

Another effect of the increase of fluids circulating in the body is a lowering of the sodium concentration, which is why you shouldn't restrict your salt intake during pregnancy (see p. 77) unless you have serious fluid retention.

HEART

With more fluids to push around the body, the heart has extra work to do. By the end of the second trimester it has increased its workload by 40 per cent. It enlarges to accommodate this extra work but astonishingly your pulse rate is hardly raised from its pre-pregnant level. Much of the circulation increase is directed to the uterus. Blood flow to the kidneys also increases as does the blood flowing through your skin, so that it is warmer and sweats more. During the third trimester, the uterus may press on the large vein in the abdomen if you lie on your back. This causes blood pressure to fall and may make you feel dizzy and faint.

LUNGS

To keep blood well supplied with oxygen, the lungs have to work harder. Take plenty of fresh air and exercise, so that the blood supply to the lungs will be improved. During the third trimester, the uterus will begin to crowd the lungs out. You may feel uncomfortable, and find yourself having to take deep breaths. Sitting up straight helps, even in bed.

KIDNEYS

Your kidneys have to filter and clean 50 per cent more blood than they did before. All renal function becomes more efficient, the body getting rid of waste products like urea and uric acid faster than before. But the kidneys don't distinguish between waste products and nutrients, so glucose is also quickly cleared from the blood, together with minerals and vitamins – for instance, water-soluble vitamin C, plus folic acid which is excreted at four or five times the usual rate. This is one of the reasons for making sure your vitamin and mineral intake is maintained during pregnancy, and why you may need folic acid supplements (see p. 77). In addition to the greater amount of urine to be got rid of, you will find you need to pass urine more often than usual as the expanding uterus irritates the neighbouring bladder. Even though it is annoying, don't restrict your fluid intake.

JOINTS

The ligaments that surround, connect and support the joints are softened and become more flexible, especially in the pelvis, due to the action of pregnancy hormones. In labour the joints of the pelvis can stretch, allowing your baby a smooth passage to the outside world. Joints affected include the sacroiliac joint, and the junction of the pubic bones at the

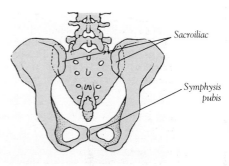

Sacroiliac

Symphysis pubis

SACROILIAC JOINT
It is located at the top of the buttocks and can be associated with low back pain.

front, the symphysis pubis. Increased fluid retention during pregnancy may cause movement of the symphysis pubis which can be painful. See a physiotherapist if you are affected by this.

After about week 16, the weight of the growing baby pushing down in the pelvis can tip the pelvic brim forward. The changed angle puts strain on the muscles and ligaments surrounding the lower spine, and may cause backache. You can counter the forward tilt with good posture and by doing pelvic tilt exercises (see p. 90). Your legs and feet may also ache. Good posture (see p. 80), exercise, shoes with some support and massage (see p. 105) can do a lot to counteract discomfort.

Skin

THOUGH SOME WOMEN DO GLOW with good health during pregnancy, there are some changes to the skin that are not so flattering, but they usually disappear shortly after the birth of the baby.

PIGMENTATION

Some degree of darkening is a universal characteristic of pregnancy, although its depth varies according to skin colour. Blondes, redheads, and even brunettes who have pale skins may see little change, whereas olive-skinned women may find that their whole skin darkens and areas like the nipples, abdomen and genital region remain dark brown after delivery.

Pigmentation of the nipples and areolas and a dark line down the centre of the abdomen, called the linea nigra, usually make their appearance around week 14. The linea nigra can be up to 1 cm (½ in) wide and stretches from the pubic hair to the navel, or even up to the breast bone. The navel tends to darken, and by the third trimester it stretches, becoming completely flat by 40 weeks. It returns to normal after delivery. The linea nigra also begins to fade shortly after delivery, but may take several months to disappear completely, or remain as a shadow.

Any brown birthmarks, moles, freckles, or recent scars, particularly on the abdomen, may darken during pregnancy. The effect becomes more obvious after exposure to sunlight, but will probably return to normal shortly after delivery. Blotchy and irregular brown patches (chloasma) sometimes appear and are made worse by sunlight (see p. 98). They usually begin to fade shortly after delivery and may disappear completely in a few months.

TEXTURE

It's impossible to anticipate whether your skin, particularly on your face, will become drier or oilier, improve or get worse during pregnancy. High levels of hormones have several effects on skin, as does the greater amount of blood circulating to it. Oiliness results from the action of progesterone, which encourages the secretion of sebum. Spots can appear unexpectedly (see p. 99) because of fluctuating hormone levels, not just on the face, but on the back too. Increased fluid retention can fill out lines or cause unwelcome puffiness (see p. 99), depending on your face shape. However, these changes are all normal and will disappear after your baby is born.

STRETCHMARKS

These occur in the skin under several different conditions. The first is in adolescence when we grow quickly. The second is whenever we put on a large amount of weight in a short time, and the third is during pregnancy. The underlying cause is always the same – tearing of collagen bundles. Collagen is the "skeleton" of the skin; its network of elastic bundles allows the skin to stretch with movement or with a change in size or shape. The marks in pregnancy are due to the high level of sex hormones that are circulating in the blood. One of the effects of these hormones is to break down and remove protein from the skin, thereby disrupting the collagen bundles and making the skin thin and papery. It appears delicate and stretchy in certain areas – the stretchmarks.

The stretchmarks that occur when we put on a lot of weight result when the collagen bundles are stretched to the point of breaking by the fat, which is laid down underneath the skin.

During pregnancy, these marks appear on the breasts, the abdomen, and also on the thighs and buttocks. They will remain pinkish throughout pregnancy, but after delivery they shrink and become a silvery colour after nine months or so.

Hair and nails

THESE ARE BOTH MADE from the same substance – keratin – and you may or may not notice any changes to your hair (see also p. 98) and fingernails.

HAIR CHANGES

Pregnancy can have an unpredictable and quite dramatic effect on hair. Curls may straighten out or straight hair become curly, and these changes can remain after your baby is born. Some women's hair becomes luxuriant and shiny, others' lifeless or greasy. Even body hair may become more or less apparent.

Most women's hair becomes more oily, particularly towards the end of the pregnancy, due to the very high levels of progesterone in the blood, which stimulate the sebaceous glands on the scalp. Dry hair may benefit from this change, though it can make hair lank. If you've always had normal hair, you may find any change difficult to live with because your hair won't be as predictable as it was before. Because of this unpredictability, pregnancy is not a good time to dye your hair or have a perm.

One reason hair may become progressively thicker is that hormonal changes cause more than 90 per cent of the hair on your head to be thrown simultaneously into a growing phase (normally only 90 per cent are growing and the remainder resting). Therefore during pregnancy, your hair should be thicker and stronger, although this will not apply to every woman.

Soon after birth the hair that you would normally lose, but didn't because of your pregnancy, will be lost in large amounts, making way for the new. Hair loss can go on for anything up to 18 months and, if replacement is too slow, the hair becomes thinner and thinner. This can be alarming, but no woman has gone bald simply as a result of pregnancy, so be assured that your hair will eventually recover.

Facial and body hair goes into a growing phase, too, which may increase its quantity and strength. Women with dark skins, in whom pregnancy causes a greatly increased amount of pigmentation, may find that their body and facial hair darkens. In some cases this hair does not return to its former colour.

NAIL CHANGES

Splitting and breaking of nails is another problem for some women in pregnancy. Use rubber gloves and hand lotion to protect the nails. They will return to normal after delivery, although those who have stronger, shinier nails in pregnancy may suffer brittleness after delivery.

Teeth and gums

It used to be said that a baby absorbed the calcium from its mother's teeth and therefore women were more susceptible to tooth decay during pregnancy than at other times. This is not so, as there is no way of extracting calcium from the teeth. However, the high levels of progesterone that are produced during pregnancy will make the margins of the gums around the teeth soft and spongy, predisposing them to infection. It is therefore essential that you are meticulous about oral hygiene and avoid the sugary foods that lead to tooth decay. Make an appointment to see your dentist as soon as you know you are pregnant and keep up your regular check-ups throughout pregnancy and lactation. Remember to tell your dentist that you are pregnant as you should avoid X-rays.

5

Emotional changes

Psychologically speaking, your main task during pregnancy is to incorporate your new baby into your long-term planning, your future, your feelings and your lifestyle. Though these challenges are similar for men and women, you can be affected differently. Any emotional turmoil you feel is a positive force to guide you through your adjustment to becoming a mother or father, helping you to be emotionally well prepared for your new baby. The fact that you may have second thoughts doesn't mean that you've made a mistake. It would be wrong to think that having a baby is all fun. The best thing you can do is to be open about your feelings. If you talk to each other honestly, you will clarify your thinking and prepare the basis for a constant exchange throughout the pregnancy.

Self-image

THE CHANGING SIZE AND SHAPE of your body may make you feel strange about yourself, and you may even worry about becoming fat or unattractive to your partner. Try to be positive about your shape. Look for the beauty in the fullness of your breasts and the curve of your abdomen. For both men and women, a pregnant body is extremely sensuous and a pregnant woman is beautiful in her own way. Your image of yourself in this condition is important. Feeling proud of your shape and your fertility will make you more positive about your condition and encourage you to take a general interest in looking good (see p. 94), being healthy (see p. 73) and keeping fit (see pp. 80–93).

HOW HORMONES AFFECT MOOD

Mood changes are largely a reflection of the tremendous change in hormonal secretions, so there's no need to feel guilty about them. The upheaval of pregnancy makes nearly all women feel emotionally fragile, prone to crying and feelings of panic. Even in the most positive of pregnancies you may feel some confusion. Once you know it's normal to feel low, you'll feel better and your moods will pass more quickly. Try not to be too analytical; react to the next thing that comes along.

YOUR CHANGING SHAPE
You should feel confident and proud of your rounded body: think of it as a reaffirmation of life.

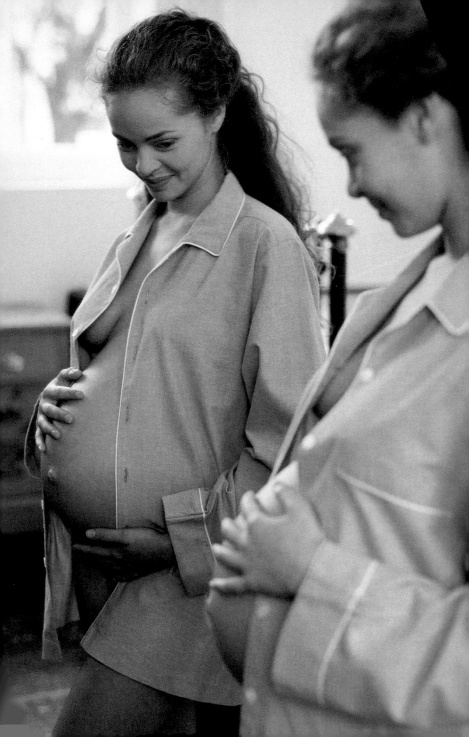

Feelings about your partner

THE CHANGE FROM BEING an individual to being a parent is one of the most profound you'll ever experience; a woman is different from a mother; a father is not the same as a man. Approaching parenthood together is an essentially positive and deeply satisfying experience but you're going to find it shattering, exhausting and incredibly hard work too.

There are going to be many ups and downs for you and your partner to cope with during pregnancy. Be prepared for them and give them time and patience. If you're in a good partnership, one of the things that you'll almost certainly feel is that the pregnancy cements your relationship. If you can, try to go away for a weekend or have a holiday when you're between four and seven months pregnant (the time when most women feel at their best), as it will give you a chance to share your feelings and help you look forward to the exciting times ahead.

The strengthening of your bonds may be a little claustrophobic at first until you get used to it. It might help if you agree from the very beginning that you'll talk about things relating to the pregnancy in an open way, and that you won't interpret your partner's comments as rejection or unkindness. During this time it's quite common for couples to make unusual demands on each other as a test of loyalty and devotion, but try to be realistic about small grievances and be quick to point them out and explain them to each other. The reality of approaching parenthood can sometimes cause tension, but this can usually be defused if you decide to be frank with each other. Friction and conflict seem to diminish when each partner is prepared to be generous towards the other.

You'll certainly start evaluating each other in the light of your new roles. You may have always had an image of the kind of parent you would want your partner to be and you'll try to see how he or she measures up to your fantasy. Don't be too hard in your evaluation of your partner; think about how you would feel by evaluating yourself in the same way. This will make you sympathetic towards your partner's feelings about being judged all the time.

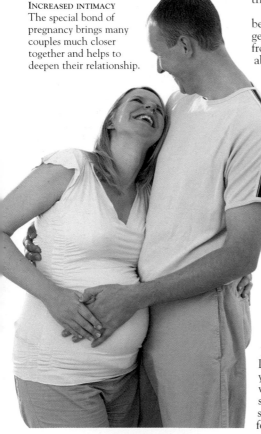

INCREASED INTIMACY
The special bond of pregnancy brings many couples much closer together and helps to deepen their relationship.

BEING AN INVOLVED FATHER

Every father needs to take an active rather than a passive role in a fundamental life event such as the birth of his child. You need to feel that you really are contributing something as well and, even better, that you're taking this important step together.

Becoming a father doesn't start with the birth of your child: it helps to get involved with your partner's pregnancy from the beginning, to understand what is going on in her body and to understand the physical and emotional pressures she is experiencing. Nearly all women are helped by the presence of their partner at the first antenatal visit, for example.

As a prospective father, you may be wondering how you can help your partner through her pregnancy while making sure that your own needs are met, but you have to be prepared for your life to be disrupted to some extent. The golden rule is to be observant of your partner's needs, to assist in her care, and to be closely linked with everything that's happening to her. Fatherhood always involves hard work, a lot of responsibility and a considerable amount of time but will repay you with immeasurable joy, satisfaction and happiness. During pregnancy, the delivery and after the birth, your partner will be depending on you for courage and support. If she doesn't get them from you she will feel alone, which is bad for her and for your baby.

It's not uncommon for a father-to-be to discover feelings of jealousy towards his partner and her condition during a first pregnancy. You may feel neglected if your partner seems more ready to share information about her pregnancy with women friends rather than with you. If you find that you are trying to minimize her requests, her problems and needs, take a look at yourself. Make a special effort to be reasonable, and listen, sympathize and encourage. She will almost certainly return your gifts, which means acceptance of you not only as lover but now also as the father of your child.

The interdependence on one another is not easy in practice and certain traditions of bringing up boys don't facilitate it. The strong, silent loner doesn't easily make an involved father. It's easier to learn from a good parent who acts as an example, but you may have to educate yourself into fatherhood by devising your own way of learning.

It may hearten you to know that mothers and fathers start off more or less equally ignorant about babies and small children. Mothers do eventually learn something out of necessity and trial and error. Unless you're involved, you'll not even be that lucky. It's a tragedy to miss out on the care of your child and instead remain a kind of stranger. Also remember that there's no one right or wrong way to be a parent, but you have to be ready to grow just as your child is growing – in caring, in admitting mistakes, and in making time available among your family members. All these things will help to make you a better father.

Special anxieties

NEARLY EVERY PROSPECTIVE parent, but particularly a mother, is beset by anxieties about the baby, especially in the last trimester. The immediacy of delivery and having a new baby nurtures natural anxieties about whether the baby will have any kind of abnormality, whether you will be a capable parent, whether you will do something silly like dropping the baby and whether you will be able to cope with the day-to-day care in the first weeks. All of these feelings are quite natural and most women harbour them. If you know that they are going to occur and are normal and natural, this will help to defuse your anxiety.

Dreams in particular can be disturbing. You may dream of mistreating your baby or not caring for it properly. You may dream of losing the baby or that it is stillborn. Your dreams represent a perfectly legitimate fear in both these respects; fear that you have at the back of your mind, but during your waking hours are not prepared to face. Think of your dreams as a release for your anxieties. The fact that you may dream about harming your baby doesn't mean that you really want to harm it or ever would; it's a healthy symptom of wanting to do the best for your baby.

Every pregnant woman at some stage worries about something being wrong with the baby. Dreaming about losing the baby or about having a stillbirth has little foundation in reality. It's more likely to do with figuratively losing the baby from your uterus. Dreams about the baby dying are part of your understandable concern for your baby's well-being. One way of dealing with them is to try to put them out of your head upon waking and get on with some pleasurable aspect of preparing for the baby's arrival.

All women worry about how they'll behave in labour. Will the pain be too much? Will they scream? Will their bowels or bladder empty embarrassingly? Will they lose control of themselves and act foolishly? Such fears are normal and the chances are you'll be surprised at how calmly you behave, though most of us do something rather silly at some time during the labour and birth. It isn't important. Remember midwives and doctors have seen it all before; you can't embarrass them.

Sex in pregnancy

THE MAJORITY OF WOMEN I have spoken to about sex and pregnancy have almost universally felt that sex was better than ever. Because of the high level of circulating hormones, a woman can become stimulated more readily and reach a high pitch of sexual excitement more quickly than in the non-pregnant state. Many parts of her body, such as the breasts, nipples and genital area (see p. 60), are more sensitive during pregnancy because all the sexual organs become highly developed and more capable of arousal than before pregnancy occurred. Also there is the freedom from having to use contraceptive methods.

There does, however, tend to be some loss of libido during the first and third trimesters. This could be a result of increased hormonal activity at the beginning of pregnancy, causing nausea and tiredness, and of your large shape at the end. Even if you don't feel like making love, and many couples don't, explore other ways of touching and giving sexual pleasure to each other.

There doesn't seem to be any medical reason why you should not enjoy full sexual intercourse throughout your pregnancy, as the womb is completely sealed off by the mucous plug. However, an article in one of Britain's medical journals entitled "Does sex embarrass the fetus?" did point out that a great deal of sexual activity might encourage maternal infections. But the report showed that this was probably related to other factors including hygiene, even possibly different sexual partners.

As long as you only have sex with your partner, and only when you feel like it, and as long as it isn't too athletic, sex is to be recommended throughout pregnancy, unless your doctor advises you otherwise or other factors relate to your condition (see opposite). Sex is good for your body too – orgasm exercises the uterine muscles, though this can cause contractions later on in pregnancy, which die down after a few minutes. Sex also helps you to become more aware of your pelvic floor muscles.

WILL SEX HARM THE BABY?

There is no information suggesting that sex harms the baby. Sex cannot introduce infection to the baby because it is safely protected in a surrounding bag of fluid. Sex will not crush the baby either. The bag of fluid (amniotic sac) is an excellent cushion and once the baby is firmly attached to its mother's uterus, there is no way that intercourse can cause a miscarriage. If the baby should miscarry it will be for reasons other than the fact you are having sexual intercourse, as will the onset of labour. Labour will not start simply because of the stimulation of sex.

WHEN NOT TO HAVE SEX

● If you have placenta praevia.
● If bleeding occurs, consult your doctor immediately and do not have sex. It may not be serious but your doctor has to rule out the possibility of placenta praevia or of miscarriage.
● If you have had a previous miscarriage, ask your doctor's advice or ask at your antenatal clinic. You may be advised to abstain during the early months while the pregnancy establishes itself.
● If you have a show (see p. 117) or the waters break, there is a risk of infection.

POSITIONS FOR INTERCOURSE DURING PREGNANCY

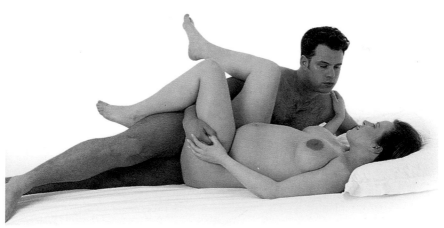

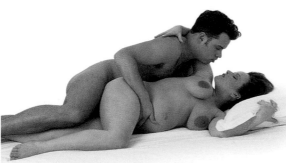

NEW POSITIONS
Your enlarging abdomen and tender breasts may make intercourse in conventional lovemaking positions uncomfortable. Trying some new positions, such as the ones shown here, may help, and ask your partner not to penetrate too deeply.

6

Health and nutrition

To ensure that your baby develops in a healthy environment, you should keep your body as fit and well nourished as you possibly can. It's not a question of devising a special diet for pregnancy, it is more to do with eating a good variety of the right foods – those that are rich in the essential nutrients. If you are deficient in any part of your diet, this may affect not only your health but also how well you can support the pregnancy and nourish the baby. You also need to be aware of the risks posed by nicotine, alcohol and drugs as they can have a detrimental effect on the growth and well-being of the baby.

Weight gain

NOWADAYS IT IS KNOWN that you should gain a lot more weight in pregnancy than was thought healthy in the past. The amount of weight put on by women in pregnancy varies between 9 and 13.5kg (20–30lb) with the most rapid gain usually between weeks 24 and 32. Your uterus, plus the baby, the placenta and the fluids will account for more than half of your total weight gain. You also manufacture more blood (see p. 60) and you lay down fat to prepare for lactation.

I would not want to encourage anyone to gain an excessive amount of weight, but dieting is not a good idea during pregnancy. It is much more important to eat a balanced and varied diet. A British study showed that there was a higher incidence of low-birthweight babies amongst those women who ate less than the recommended levels of calories, vitamins and minerals.

On the other hand, there is a lower incidence of physical and mental abnormalities, spontaneous abortions and neonatal deaths when mothers have relatively high weight gain (though not when they become obese) and babies are born heavier. It has also been shown that prolonged labours are directly related to the way in which the uterus has grown during pregnancy, and that in turn depends on how well nourished the mother has been.

EATING WELL
A balanced diet that includes plenty of fresh fruit and vegetables will keep you healthy during pregnancy.

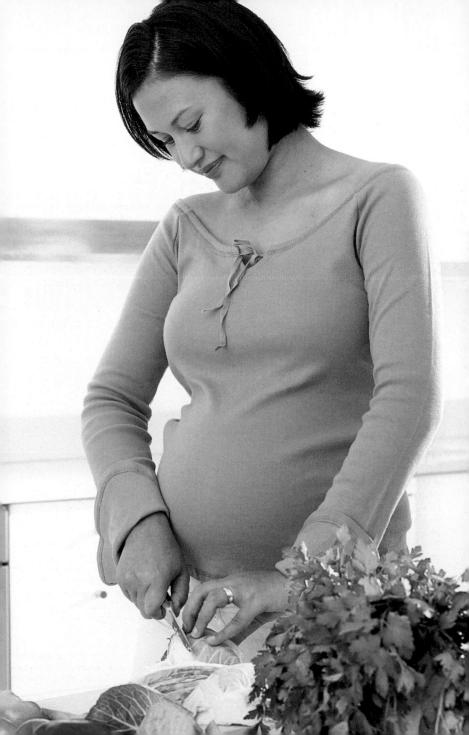

WHAT YOU GAIN

Rather than emphasizing restriction, nowadays doctors consider that minimum weight gain for most women should be 11kg (24lb). When a woman eats what she needs, her weight gain usually follows a natural and predictable pattern. You may find you put on weight and your figure changes almost from the time you confirm the pregnancy (6–8 weeks). However, your weight gain may be monitored from about 12 weeks at your antenatal checks.

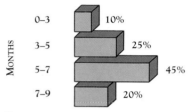

MONTHS

0–3	10%
3–5	25%
5–7	45%
7–9	20%

PERCENTAGE OF TOTAL WEIGHT GAIN
This is a rough guide to your weight gain at a given time during pregnancy.

BEING OVERWEIGHT

Although there is no ideal weight gain to aim for, it's still not a good idea for weight gain to be excessive. True obesity presents problems: it puts extra strain on the heart, which is already working at full stretch, and there is an association between excessive weight gain and Caesarean section. It's thought that when fat accumulates between the muscle fibres of the uterus they work less efficiently and cannot contract enough to finish pushing the baby out once labour has started.

If you're definitely overweight and have been trying to lose weight, it's important that you stop dieting when you decide to try for a baby. Unless your doctor considers you are dangerously obese, choose your foods with care when you're trying to conceive and once you are pregnant, but don't do anything drastic about losing weight until you have finished breastfeeding your baby.

AWARENESS OF WEIGHT GAIN

If you run to plumpness during pregnancy, fat has a tendency to accumulate in places such as the thighs and upper arms. It is sometimes extremely difficult to lose this fat again after the birth. As this is demoralizing, here are a few tips to help you keep your weight gain within reasonable limits.

● As soon as you know that you are pregnant, get someone to take a snapshot of you, and take one every month or so after that. This reminder of your changing shape will help you keep your size in perspective, and if you feel you might be putting on too much weight, it may help you to combat cravings for foods with a high fat or sugar content.

● If you've always had a tendency to weight problems, but managed to keep them under control, it's easy to relapse into over-eating once you know you're pregnant. Start eating sensibly from the beginning; try not to over-eat in the first trimester when your appetite will almost certainly increase, even if you suffer from nausea some of the time.

● Try to eat regular, nutritious meals, and eat little and often when your pregnancy is more advanced. You're less likely to feel hungry in between.

● Keep a supply of nutritious snacks – cheese, fresh and dried fruit, wholemeal rolls – in the house and at your place of work at all times. Avoid the high-calorie, low-nutrition foods that are so accessible, such as candy bars, crisps and fizzy drinks.

● When preparing meals or snacks, follow these simple rules: eat unprocessed foods; include lots of roughage in your diet; grill rather than fry foods; sweeten with natural sweeteners.

● Don't eat as a way of cheering yourself up. If thinking about your baby and the birth makes you too distracted to concentrate on any serious project that would normally occupy you, at least have a project such as a jigsaw puzzle or a piece of embroidery to break up your routine.

GUIDELINES FOR EATING

Most of the daily food guides for pregnant women, with long lists of items to be prepared and measured out, don't take into account how busy most women are, or that they may not always be at home for meals. Rather than worry about exact portions, or lists, you should understand why you need certain foods and nutrients and work out your own plan for healthy eating. If you suffer from nausea, you may also have to plan when to prepare meals.

WHAT TO EAT

Your appetite will increase and by the fourth month of your pregnancy you may feel hungry all the time. This is nature's way of making sure that you take enough food for yourself and the baby. This doesn't mean you can "eat for two". It's perfectly normal to eat more as your metabolism speeds up, but your energy requirements increase only by about 15 per cent, which means that 500 extra calories a day will be sufficient.

Every bit of food you take in should be good for you and the baby. If you ate well before you became pregnant, you should be healthy enough to get through any period of nausea. As your pregnancy progresses, try eating a greater number of smaller meals; small, frequent meals are always more easily digested. Bowel contractions slow down during pregnancy so the stomach empties more slowly and should not be overloaded at any one time. Your developing baby pushes up into your stomach during the last trimester, constricting its capacity, so a small meal is more easily accommodated and you'll feel more comfortable. The problem then arises of what sort of foods to eat as snacks. Avoid crisps and biscuits, which are usually low in goodness and high in calories. Be inventive, try sandwiches, nuts, fruit and soups.

FOODS TO AVOID

As a general rule, foods have a higher nutritional value the less they are processed and cooked. Choose fresh, raw wholefoods wherever you can. When planning what to eat, remember:
- Processed foods with added preservatives and colourings contain high levels of undesirable chemicals.
- White flour products or anything with added sugars provide little nutrition at the price of a lot of calories. Look at the list of ingredients on the labels of processed foods – you may be surprised how many apparently savoury foods actually contain sugar!
- Sweet fizzy drinks – even if you choose the low calorie versions – are not good for you as they provide few nutrients and may contain harmful additives.
- Strong coffee and tea adversely affect the digestive system; tannic acid in tea drunk with a meal can reduce iron absorption. Excess caffeine and tannic acid may not be good for the baby.

- Certain foods may harbour dangerous bacteria and should be avoided during pregnancy: pâté and soft cheeses (listeria), raw eggs (salmonella).
- Liver or liver products should be eaten in moderation (see p. 76).
- Undercooked meat, unpasteurized goat's milk and goat's milk products may contain a parasite called toxoplasma, which can seriously harm the unborn baby. Only eat meat that has been cooked thoroughly. Avoid unpasteurized goat's milk and goat's milk products.
- Wash all fruits and vegetables thoroughly before eating or cooking to remove any traces of soil.
- Certain moulds produce toxic substances so avoid eating fruits and vegetables with diseased skins, or any foods that are very mouldy, or dried foods that are stale. It is not enough to remove the mouldy parts as the harmful substances can penetrate deeper and they will not be destroyed by cooking.

Vital nutrients needed in pregnancy

YOU SHOULDN'T NEED to eat more food than you did before you were pregnant, but you should be aware of the nutrients present in the foods you choose to eat.

PROTEIN

Your protein requirements increase by about 50 per cent when you are pregnant. In one day sufficient protein could be gained from three eggs, ½ litre (1 pint) milk, 100g (¼ lb) cheese, or a good helping of fish or lean meat. These foods all contain the essential amino acids (the chemical substances that make up protein). Vegetable proteins contain only some of the amino acids so they need to be combined with animal protein or some wheat products to make them complete protein (see below). Vegetable proteins are found in peas, beans and lentils, brewer's yeast, seeds and nuts.

CALORIES

During pregnancy you will need about 500 more calories a day than the usual requirement of 2000–2500. You will need even more calories if you're having a baby within a short time of a previous one, or if you are still working, busy looking after a family, underweight or under stress. You shouldn't have to concentrate deliberately on calorie-counting – most women are too busy to do this anyway – you will get sufficient calories if you eat a varied diet.

FIBRE AND FLUIDS

As pregnancy progresses there is a tendency to develop constipation. You can help to overcome it by giving your intestines plenty of roughage to work on. Raw fruit and vegetables, bran, wholegrains, peas and beans are all fibrous foods that you should eat some of every day.

You should not regulate your fluid intake during pregnancy, except to watch the calorie content of the drinks you take. Water is the best drink, helping to keep your kidneys working well and to avoid constipation. If you do suffer from mild fluid retention (oedema), you won't affect your condition by reducing your fluid intake.

VEGETARIAN DIET

Achieving a balanced diet with sufficient quantities of protein and all the vitamins and minerals doesn't require any more effort if you are a vegetarian. There are plant sources of protein that are complementary, so if you eat foods in combination you will gain all the necessary amino acids (see above). For example, if you are eating grains – rice or corn – combine them with dried beans or peas or nuts. If your meal is made up of fresh vegetables, add a few sesame seeds, nuts or mushrooms to supply the missing amino acids. Few people eat one food in isolation anyway. There is relatively little iron in each helping of plant food, even leafy green vegetables and beans, and

these foods often contain substances that interfere with the body's absorption of iron, so vegetarians need to make sure that they eat plenty of foods that contain iron.

Pregnant vegetarians who don't take any dairy products (vegans) will need to be a little more careful that their diet is rich in foods that contain calcium, Vitamin D (or get plenty of sunshine) and riboflavin. The most difficult problem is adequate intake of Vitamin B_{12} which is only found in animal sources. Very little is needed but lack of it will lead to a form of anaemia. It can be prepared commercially from fungi and you should consult your doctor about taking this synthetic B_{12} if you are vegan.

VITAMINS

The value of a varied and balanced diet of wholesome food is that you will take in high enough levels of vitamins without resorting to vitamin supplements. Research has shown, however, that multivitamin supplements, if taken before conception and during the first trimester, can prevent neural tube defects such as anencephaly and spina bifida. There are other women who doctors consider may benefit from supplements (see below).

MINERALS

You are not likely to be deficient in minerals and trace elements if you eat a good diet. However, calcium and iron intakes need to be maintained and some doctors and clinics routinely prescribe dietary supplements of iron and folic acid. If supplements are not provided, ask if you need any. Your doctor may have assessed your diet and decided that it will be sufficient. Don't medicate yourself with supplements without your doctor knowing; discuss this with him or her first. Women who are nutritionally vulnerable, however, will certainly benefit from appropriate supplementation.

CALCIUM

A sufficient quantity of about twice your pre-pregnant intake is important from the time of conception because your baby's teeth and bones begin to form from weeks 4–6. As your baby grows, so your calcium requirements increase – by week 25 they have more than doubled. Sources of calcium include dairy foods, leafy vegetables, dried peas, beans and lentils, and nuts. Calcium cannot be absorbed efficiently without Vitamin D. However, this vitamin is not found in great quantities in many foods and the best source is sunlight. The body can make its own Vitamin D with the help of the sun so you don't need to worry about eating foods rich in Vitamin D (butter, milk, egg yolk) unless you never expose your skin to sunlight.

Calcium supplements will be useful if you are allergic to cow's milk. You will need up to 1200mg daily in a compound form, although if you eat well, 600mg should be sufficient. Vitamin D will also be prescribed and is usually given in the form of halibut oil capsules which contain Vitamin A as well.

IRON

The large increase in blood volume means that extra iron is needed to make haemoglobin for the increased number of red blood cells. The more haemoglobin the blood contains, the more oxygen it can carry to the various tissues, including the placenta. Your iron reserves will also be needed by the baby to have in reserve for after the birth, because breast milk contains only traces of iron.

Iron is quite difficult for the body to absorb. That from animal sources (prawns, egg yolk) is more easily absorbed than

NUTRITIONALLY VULNERABLE WOMEN

If any of the following apply to you, you need to make a special effort to eat well during pregnancy and will almost certainly need supplements to maintain your health and the general health of your baby.

- You are allergic to certain key foods, such as cow's milk or wheat.
- Before conception you were generally run-down, underweight or eating a poor and unbalanced diet.
- You have had a recent miscarriage or stillbirth, or your children are spaced closely together.
- You drink or smoke heavily.
- You have a chronic condition that obliges you to take some form of medication constantly.
- You are adolescent and still growing.
- You have a multiple pregnancy.
- For reasons beyond your control you have to work particularly hard or are subject to a lot of stress.

that in whole grains and nuts, but eating foods rich in Vitamin C at the same time as those that are iron-rich can double the amount of iron absorbed.

If women are iron-deficient when they become pregnant or develop a deficiency later on, iron tablets may be prescribed to prevent anaemia developing (see p. 45).

There has been much unnecessary alarm about one iron-rich foodstuff, liver (and liver products). This is because cattle feeds are usually rich in Vitamin A, which is concentrated in the animal's liver. Excessively large doses of Vitamin A may carry a small risk to the baby of birth defects, so you should eat liver no more than once a week, in a small portion.

If you suffer from indigestion and take medication, be careful about your iron intake; antacid medicines limit iron absorption. Also, be aware that food cooked in iron pots absorbs iron, increasing the food's iron content by some three to 30 times.

VITAMINS AND MINERALS REQUIRED IN PREGNANCY

NAME	FOOD SOURCE	WHAT IT DOES
VITAMIN A (retinol)	whole milk, fortified margarine, butter, egg yolk, oily fish, fish liver oils, liver, kidneys, green and yellow vegetables, carrots – cooking the carrots releases Vitamin A for easy absorption	Builds up resistance to infection, essential for good vision, keeps skin and mucous membranes in good condition, necessary for the formation of tooth enamel, hair and fingernails, important for the growth and formation of the thyroid gland.
VITAMIN B$_1$ (thiamine)	whole grains, nuts, pulses, liver, heart, kidneys, brewer's yeast, wheatgerm – don't overcook, benefits will be lost	Aids digestion, keeps the stomach and intestine healthy, needed for fertility, growth and lactation; the body's needs increase during illness and infection.
VITAMIN B$_2$ (riboflavin)	brewer's yeast, wheatgerm, whole grains, green vegetables, milk, eggs, liver – goodness can be lost if foods are exposed to light	Helps break down all food, prevents eye and skin problems, essential at the time of conception and early in pregnancy for normal development of the embryo.
NIACIN (B$_3$)	brewer's yeast, whole grains, liver, wheatgerm, green vegetables, oily fish, kidneys, eggs, milk, peanuts	Builds brain cells, prevents infections and bleeding of the gums.
PANTOTHENIC ACID (B$_5$)	liver, kidneys, heart, eggs, peanuts, wheatbran, whole grains, cheese	Essential for all normal reproductive functions of the body, maintains red blood cells.
VITAMIN B$_6$ (pyridoxine)	brewer's yeast, whole grains, liver, heart, kidneys, wheatgerm, mushrooms, potatoes, bananas, molasses, dried vegetables	Helps the body to assimilate fats and fatty acids necessary for the production of antibodies which fight disease; deficiency causes disease of the nerves and anaemia.
VITAMIN B$_{12}$ (cyanocobalamin)	liver, brewer's yeast, wheatgerm, whole grains, milk, soya beans, fish	Essential for the development of healthy red blood cells, necessary for the formation of the baby's central nervous system.
FOLIC ACID (one of B complex)	raw leaf vegetables, lamb's liver, walnuts	Essential for blood formation, helps to prevent neural tube defects, such as spina bifida; essential for the development of the central nervous system.

FOLIC ACID

Folic acid is essential for the supply of nucleic acids needed by the dividing cells of the embryo. As the body can't store folic acid and in pregnancy excretes four or five times the normal amount, enough must be eaten every day. Folic acid is found in leafy vegetables and nuts, but folic acid supplements should ideally be taken for three months before you become pregnant and throughout pregnancy.

Supplements of higher doses up to 4mg may be prescribed for women who have previously had babies with brain and spinal cord defects such as spina bifida.

SALT

Ordinarily most of us take in too much sodium, but while you are pregnant, maintain a sensible salt intake. Any excess salt in your blood is diluted during pregnancy by the increase in body fluids.

NAME	FOOD SOURCE	WHAT IT DOES
VITAMIN C (ascorbic acid)	citrus fruits, fresh fruit, red, green and yellow vegetables – destroyed by overcooking	Helps resistance to infection, builds a strong placenta, helps the absorption of iron from the intestine, a useful detoxicant in the body, important for the repair of fractures and wound healing. Needs are variable; infection, fever and stress deplete the body's resources and needs increase.
VITAMIN D (calciferol)	fortified milk, oily fish, liver oils, butter, egg yolk – sunshine activates a previtamin in the skin (see p. 75)	Promotes the absorption of calcium from the intestine and helps the incorporation of calcium from the blood and tissues into bone cells to strengthen the bones.
VITAMIN E	wheatgerm, most other foods	Necessary for the healthy maintenance of cell membranes, also helps protect certain fatty acids.
VITAMIN K	green leafy vegetables – manufactured by the body from bacteria in the gut	Helps in the process by which blood coagulates.
CALCIUM	milk, hard cheese, whole small fish, peanuts, walnuts, sunflower seeds, green vegetables	Essential for the formation of healthy bones and teeth, important in the early months when the baby's teeth are developing.
IRON	kidneys, liver, shellfish, egg yolks, red meat, molasses, apricots, haricot beans, raisins, prunes	Essential for healthy formation of the red blood cells.
ZINC	wheatbran, eggs, liver, nuts, onions, shellfish, sunflower seeds, wheatgerm, whole wheat	Helps in formation of many enzymes (special proteins that oversee chemical reactions in our bodies) and of proteins, needed to ensure the release of Vitamin A from liver stores into the bloodstream.

Dangerous substances

IF YOU NORMALLY SMOKE or drink, you should change your habits during pregnancy to protect your unborn baby. You also need to be meticulous about hygiene, particularly when handling raw meat and when cleaning out cat litter. Raw meat and cat faeces contain a parasite, toxoplasma, that can damage your unborn child.

SMOKING

● The chemicals absorbed from cigarette smoke limit fetal growth by reducing the number of cells produced, both in the baby's body and brain. Nicotine makes blood vessels constrict and therefore reduces the blood supply to the placenta, interfering with the nourishment of the baby.
● The level of carbon monoxide is higher in a smoker's blood, and whatever the level in the woman's blood it's higher in the baby's blood. As well as being a poison, carbon monoxide reduces the amount of oxygen that blood can carry. The more carbon monoxide in the baby's blood, the lower its weight at birth. The babies of mothers who smoke can be as much as 200g (7oz) lighter than those of mothers who don't smoke, and low birthweight babies can have problems and are less likely to survive. The incidence of prematurity almost doubles in smokers.
● Studies have shown that smokers are more likely to have children with all types of congenital malformations, especially cleft palate, hare lip and central nervous system abnormalities, with the risk more than doubled in heavy smokers.
● Smokers have nearly twice the risk of spontaneous abortion (miscarriage and stillbirth), partly because smoking greatly increases the risk of the placenta being attached too low down in the uterus, and partly because smokers' placentas tend to be thinner and age prematurely.
● Neonatal deaths are more common among babies whose mothers smoked.

Mothers who continue to smoke after the fourth month are increasing by nearly one third the risk of their baby dying.
● The effects of smoking in pregnancy last for a long time after your baby is born, and children who live in smoking households are less healthy than others in many respects. Exposure to cigarette smoke puts babies at considerable risk during the first year of life – they have a tendency to develop bronchitis and the incidence of cot deaths increases.

DANGERS OF SMOKING

All smoking is dangerous for your unborn child. Women who cut down on cigarettes or stop smoking before week 20 tend to

SMOKING AND PREGNANCY

Here are some of the facts about smoking and pregnancy.
● Ideally stop smoking three months before trying to conceive – men and women.
● If you need to feel something in your mouth, chew sugar-free gum (try to avoid sucking sweets or eating more.
● If you smoke when you're pregnant you risk harming your unborn baby, having a miscarriage or giving birth to an underweight baby who is vulnerable to infections.
● The children of fathers who smoke 20 or more cigarettes a day have a higher risk of cancer than children of non-smoking fathers. Smoking damages sperm, so prospective fathers should give up smoking.
● Smoking increases the likelihood of cot death.
● Once your baby is born, don't let anyone smoke while holding her (to lessen the risk of cot death.
● No one should smoke in a house where there is a baby or young child.

have babies of a similar birthweight as nonsmokers, but that still leaves the risk of congenital abnormality caused by smoking in the early stages, or even before conception. The only safe option is to give up smoking before you conceive. Women who live with smokers or are often in a smoky environment are at risk even if they never smoke themselves. Children of fathers who smoke heavily are twice as likely to have malformations.

It's particularly important that a woman who is in need of special care during pregnancy for any reason doesn't smoke because she is adding a factor that increases the possibility of something going wrong. So, if a woman has suffered a stillbirth, it is crucial that she doesn't smoke the next time she becomes pregnant as this would multiply her chances of another stillbirth.

DRINKING ALCOHOL

The extent to which alcohol, a poison, can seriously damage a developing baby has only been appreciated in the last ten or so years. Some of the alcohol of every drink you take reaches your baby's bloodstream and is most harmful during the critical development period of weeks 6–12, although each affected growth period seems to produce its own abnormalities.

There is no safe level of alcohol consumption in pregnancy. If you have more than two drinks a day, there is a 1 in 10 chance that your baby will have fetal alcohol syndrome (FAS), which can lead to facial abnormalities such as cleft palate and hare lip, heart defects, abnormal limb development and lower than average intelligence. Seriously affected babies never catch up mentally or physically with their counterparts. Binge-drinking can cause the same damage, even if you drink little as a rule: one incident of excessive alcohol consumption is just as capable of giving rise to FAS as drinking excessively all through pregnancy. You should, therefore, limit yourself to two glasses of

spirits or wine, or 570ml (1 pint) of beer on any one day. Some studies show that babies can be affected in less severe ways by intakes below two glasses a day. Perhaps this is because some mothers metabolize alcohol into poisonous acetaldehyde very quickly, perhaps because some babies are genetically less resistant to the effects of alcohol – as yet no one knows. It has been demonstrated that as little as one drink a day can double the risk of having a small-for-dates baby, and babies of women drinking half that amount tend to be shorter than expected. It is beginning to be thought that very small intakes of alcohol can cause many mental conditions so far unexplained, or affect babies mentally and physically in subtle ways. In the present state of knowledge, it would seem sensible for women once they decide to have a child, not to drink at all and to abstain from drinking alcohol throughout the pregnancy.

DRUGS

It's well known that certain drugs can affect the development of a baby, particularly at the sensitive period between weeks 6 and 12 when all the vital organs are being formed. In addition a drug may be safe in itself, but it can be harmful to the fetus if taken in combination with another equally innocent drug or certain foods.

Because of these dangers no drug of any kind, and that includes aspirin, should be taken unless under the supervision of a doctor. Don't take over-the-counter remedies for anything, or use leftover prescription drugs, or accept drugs prescribed for other people. And don't consult a doctor about anything without informing him or her that you are pregnant or trying to become pregnant.

Some drugs have to be taken for the treatment of chronic complaints such as diabetes, heart disease, thyroid problems, rheumatic disorders and possibly epilepsy, but discuss the continuation of medication with your doctor before you conceive.

7

Exercise

Both before and during pregnancy, exercise is essential. Before pregnancy, it ensures that your body is fit to carry a healthy baby to term. Once pregnant, it strengthens muscles to protect your joints and spine, which slacken prior to labour and ache when over-used. Specific exercises, when combined with breathing and relaxation techniques, help conserve energy in labour, while others prepare you for delivery positions.

Being aware of your body

YOUR BODY CHANGES in many ways during pregnancy. There are the obvious physical changes (see pp. 54–63), as well as the loosening up and stretching of the ligaments around the joints. But more important, on a day-to-day basis, is the difference in what your body can do with ease compared to what it could do before.

In later pregnancy you become a rather ungainly shape and lose some agility and mobility, becoming breathless more easily. Your centre of gravity is further forward and you are less stable. Once committed to a certain direction you may find it hard to change, and if someone bumps into you, you may fall over. To compensate for this lack of stability, you might hold your shoulders back, stand with your feet apart, and walk with a waddling gait.

These compensatory actions mean that you are using muscles in a different way and may therefore suffer minor aches and pains as pregnancy progresses. If, however, you keep your body fit during pregnancy, and protect it from stresses and strains, the muscles, joints and ligaments will take the strain more easily, without aching. You may even avoid minor discomforts

altogether. Get used to thinking that your body is in a special, not an abnormal, state, and develop reflexes and postures that take account of its needs. If you do feel uncomfortable, ease your discomfort with relaxation techniques (see p. 103).

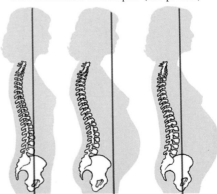

CORRECTING BAD POSTURE
Your centre of gravity (left) is affected by the growing baby in pregnancy when there is a tendency to lean back to compensate for the increased weight (centre). Good posture (right) corrects your balance and helps avoid aches.

BENDING AND LIFTING

The hormones of pregnancy soften the ligaments of the lower back and pelvis so heavy lifting should be avoided. You must protect your spine at this time and avoid unnecessary strain on your lower back when bending or lifting.

Make use of your thigh muscles when lifting. Squat down first, keeping your back straight. Prepare your body (keep your feet slightly apart) by tensing the abdominal muscles, pulling up your pelvic floor muscles (see p. 84), taking a deep breath and counting to three before lifting on four. As you lift, breathe out. Stand close to whatever you are lifting and keep it close to your body as you pick it up.
● When you are carrying anything, avoid swivelling to either side and try to distribute the weight evenly, as for instance with heavy shopping baskets.
● When you are carrying your toddler keep your body straight, don't twist, and change him from side to side.
● If you have to do anything that involves being low down, squat (see p. 91) or get down on all fours. This is a comfortable position, particularly if you do suffer from backache, as it takes the weight of the uterus off your spine.

If you have bad posture, or your back isn't flexible, improve your suppleness by sitting cross-legged against a wall. Lengthen your spine, and tilt your pelvis, pressing your back into the wall. This helps to strengthen your spine and shows you how to hold yourself well.
● Avoid lifting anything heavy down from a height. Your back will arch and you could lose your balance if the object is heavier than you supposed.

PROTECTING YOUR SPINE

In later pregnancy you will need to adapt all your movements, even basic everyday ones like getting up from lying down or getting out of a chair. You want to put the least strain possible on your back and let your thighs do the work.

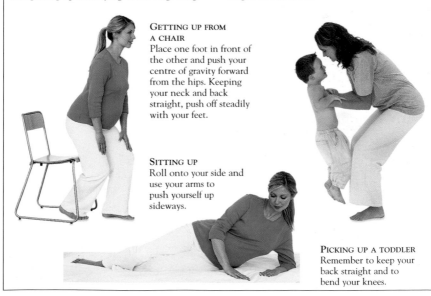

GETTING UP FROM A CHAIR
Place one foot in front of the other and push your centre of gravity forward from the hips. Keeping your neck and back straight, push off steadily with your feet.

SITTING UP
Roll onto your side and use your arms to push yourself up sideways.

PICKING UP A TODDLER
Remember to keep your back straight and to bend your knees.

Keeping active

PREGNANCY, LABOUR AND DELIVERY will make great demands on your body, so the more you can prepare yourself physically, the better. Whether you do this by continuing to exercise in the way you did before pregnancy (see p. 92) or whether you embark on a new form of exercise is up to you. The important thing is to keep yourself active. The fitter you are, the less likelihood there will be of your stiffening up as pregnancy progresses. If you make sure that you sit, stand and walk in the correct ways (see p. 81), you should avoid the aches and pains that invariably come with bad posture.

THE BENEFITS OF BEING FIT

Regular exercise will improve your mental as well as your physical well-being. Exercise causes the body to release tranquillizing chemicals, helping you to relax and soothing away tensions and anxiety. And the fast circulation of the blood that occurs when you exercise means that your body and your baby are well oxygenated.

Labour will almost certainly be easier and more comfortable if you have good muscle tone, and many of the exercises taught in antenatal classes, combined with relaxation and breathing techniques, will help give you more control over what is happening to you.

Keeping in condition during pregnancy will also mean that you regain your normal shape more quickly after delivery, and regular exercise of the pelvic floor muscles (see p. 85) will not only assist in delivery, but will also allow the muscles to regain their normal strength more quickly.

However, before you start on any exercise programme in early pregnancy, check with your doctor to make sure it is safe. Some doctors feel that if a woman has a history of miscarriage or there are any complications she should not undertake exercises in the first three months of pregnancy.

When you have the "all-clear", here are a few tips for keeping fit:
● Try to enrol in an exercise class specially designed for pregnant women. Many women find it easier to exercise regularly this way as they have the discipline of a teacher putting them through the exercises. It also helps to have someone watching you, correcting the way in which the exercises are done.
● If you haven't been an active person before pregnancy you're unlikely to change dramatically during it, but at least try to walk whenever you can, 20 minutes a day if you can manage it.
● Even if you have to sit down all day, there are exercises that you can do in a chair (see p. 89).
● Get into the habit of going through a 10–15 minute exercise programme every day. During pregnancy, exercises should be regular and taken at a slow pace. They should be rhythmic whenever possible, so it's a good idea to exercise to music.
● Always warm up gently before you start your exercise programme (see p. 86).
● Try not to go for periods with no exercise at all. Even a little exercise several times a day is better than a big burst followed by a long gap.
● Never exercise to the point of fatigue.
● Never do an exercise that causes you pain. Pain is a signal that something is wrong. Try a simpler variation of the exercise. Work towards a position gradually, don't strain.
● Try not to point your toes for too long when you're exercising as it may cause cramps in the legs.
● Most exercises are done on the floor and you might like to have a few pillows or cushions as aids to make yourself comfortable.
● Before each exercise, try a few deep breaths. This is relaxing, it makes you feel alert, it gets the blood flowing around your body and gives all your muscles a good supply of oxygen.

Antenatal exercise classes

A VARIETY OF ANTENATAL exercise classes are available and it is worth doing some research into what they have to offer and what type of teaching you'd be happiest with. The hospital or clinic will run classes (see p. 43) or you can go to an independent organization or a workshop specially for pregnant women (see p. 154 for addresses of organizations).

WHAT THEY TEACH

Some classes are run just like an ordinary exercise class, giving a thorough physical workout with exercises specifically designed for pregnant women to increase flexibility, strength and stamina. Others are designed with a certain philosophy of birth in mind. If you want to give birth in a squatting position, there will be exercises to strengthen the back and thighs, for example. The classes are also good places for making contact with other pregnant women.

MIND AND BODY
Relaxation techniques and yoga exercises prepare you both mentally and physically for the birth by keeping you supple and fit and improving breathing techniques.

YOGA

With its emphasis on muscular control of the body, breathing, relaxation and tranquillity of mind, yoga is an excellent method to use as a preparation for pregnancy. However, yoga is a philosophy which pervades the whole of life and, though special exercises for pregnancy exist, they are only a small part of the system. If you are already a devotee or have made the effort to become familiar with yoga-based exercises prior to your pregnancy, yoga can be of great help in increasing your sense of well-being.

Yoga exercises are comparable with some of those taught in antenatal classes but the types of breathing used are different. It is believed that these breathing techniques help to raise the pain threshold.

The pelvic floor muscles

THE MUSCLES THAT MAKE UP the pelvic floor support the uterus, bowel and bladder, rather like a sling holding the pelvic organs in place. They lie in two main groups, forming a figure of eight around the urethra, vagina and anus. The muscle fibres originate front and back from high up on the pubic and sacral bones. The layers of muscle overlap and are therefore thickest at the perineum.

THE ACTION OF PROGESTERONE

The pregnancy hormone progesterone prepares the body for birth by softening joints and ligaments, and that includes the pelvic floor muscles. If pressure from the enlarging uterus causes the pelvic floor to become weak, this can lead to vague aches and fatigue, to urinary incontinence and leakage, and possibly, at worst, even to prolapse of the uterus after childbirth. About half the women who have had children subsequently suffer from some weakness of the pelvic floor. As a result they may experience discomfort or so-called "stress" incontinence – slight leakage of urine when they laugh, cough, sneeze, or lift.

To counter this, a set of exercises to strengthen the pelvic floor muscles has been developed by physiotherapists working in the area of childbirth. They are known as the Kegel exercises, after Dr Arnold Kegel of the University of California in Los Angeles, one of the first physicians to recognize how important these muscles are.

Pelvic floor exercises are recommended for all women. It's best to begin doing the exercises before pregnancy and continue afterwards (they are probably even more important in older women). If you possibly can, make the exercises (see opposite) part of your daily routine.

When exercising, do about five contractions of five seconds each. Once you've mastered the exercises, you can do them wherever you are – sitting at home, standing in a queue or walking – but do remember to practise as often as you can. They will also be useful in the second stage of labour when the baby's head is about to be born (see opposite below).

LOCATING THE PELVIC FLOOR MUSCLES

Lie down with a pillow under your head and one under your knees. Cross one leg over the other and squeeze your legs tightly together. Tighten the buttock muscles and pull up as if you feel the need to empty your bladder but must wait. This helps you to locate the pelvic floor muscles, which you will feel tighten inside your vagina.

Another way to locate the muscles is to interrupt the flow midstream when you pass urine, because the muscles that control the flow of urine are your pelvic floor muscles. Only do this to find out where the muscles are and always empty your bladder completely afterwards. When doing the exercises (see opposite), ignore the abdominal and buttock muscles and use only those of the pelvic floor.

ISOLATING THE SPHINCTER MUSCLES

Lie down as above but with your legs relaxed and not crossed. Place a clean fingertip on the opening of your vagina and contract your pelvic floor muscles. You will be able to feel the contraction of the vaginal sphincter. The sphincter at the opening of the urethra is more difficult to isolate than the pelvic floor muscles because of its proximity to the vagina. But the sphincter muscles are also tightened when you contract the pelvic floor muscles. Now place your finger at the opening of your bowels and, with a larger movement, contract the muscle around the anus. You will feel the anal sphincter tightening.

STRENGTHENING THE PELVIC FLOOR

During pregnancy, the increase in the hormone progesterone causes the pelvic floor muscles to soften and relax. Here are three basic Kegel exercises which will help you to strengthen your pelvic floor muscles and keep them well toned during pregnancy. You should try to make these exercises part of your daily routine before, as well as during, pregnancy and then start them again as soon as possible after the delivery to minimize the risk of prolapse.

Contract and release

Lie on your back with your legs apart. Draw up the pelvic floor muscles, concentrating hard on the muscles of the vaginal sphincter. Hold this position for two to three seconds and then completely relax. You can try to slacken the muscles a little more and notice the release in tension. Do three of these contractions in succession.

The lift

Imagine the pelvic floor is a lift, stopping at various levels in a department store. Aim to contract the muscles gradually in five stages with a short stop at each level, not letting go between levels. Then allow the pelvic floor to descend, releasing the contraction level by level. When you reach the starting point, ground level, allow the pelvic floor muscles to relax completely so that you feel a slight bulging downwards. If you actually push downwards below this level, as if sending the lift into the basement, you can lower the pelvic floor even further, and the vaginal lips will open slightly. To do this, however, you need to hold your breath or blow out and then you should be able to feel the lips of the vagina opening. Remember, this is the position in which your pelvic floor should be if you have an internal examination and while your baby's head is being born.

During sex

Grip your partner's penis with your vagina. Hold for a few seconds before releasing. Repeat this exercise a couple of times. Your partner will be able to tell you how hard you are squeezing and will know when the strength of the squeeze is diminishing. If your partner says that he can't feel much, then you will know that you must keep exercising your pelvic muscles.

PREPARING FOR THE BIRTH OF THE BABY'S HEAD

Having an increased awareness of the pelvic floor muscles and how they feel when relaxed will help prepare you for the birth of your baby's head.

Exercise one

Lie on a bed with your knees bent, feet together and your back supported. Press your knees together hard and tighten the pelvic floor muscles at the same time. Note the feeling of tension along the inner thighs and between your legs; many women involuntarily tense these muscles when their baby's head is stretching the outlet of the birth canal, and in fact you should try to avoid this because you are more likely to tense up during delivery. Relax, and notice carefully the different feel of the muscles; this open feeling is what you should aim for when giving birth.

Exercise two

Lie on a bed, your back supported, but with your feet and knees apart. Gradually relax your thighs and pelvic floor muscles so that your knees fall wider and wider apart (your feet will roll gently onto their outer edges). At first this may seem somewhat unnatural and uncomfortable but after a little practice you will get the correct feeling of letting go fully. Practise panting in this position as you will be asked to do this by the midwife when it is time for your baby's head to pass slowly and gently out of the birth canal.

Stretching

ALWAYS PRECEDE your exercise programme by warming up with these few stretching exercises. They gently warm up muscles and joints so that you can move more freely, reducing the risk of overstretching and damage. Warming up before exercising will also reduce the risk of suffering from stiffness and cramp. Furthermore, these exercises help to stimulate the circulation, giving you

and your baby a good supply of oxygen. Repeat each exercise five to ten times; work on a firm surface, make sure you are comfortable and that your posture is good with your back straight. If necessary, lean your back against a wall or use cushions for extra support. Remembering to breathe normally throughout, start the routine slowly and if you feel any pain, discomfort or fatigue, stop at once.

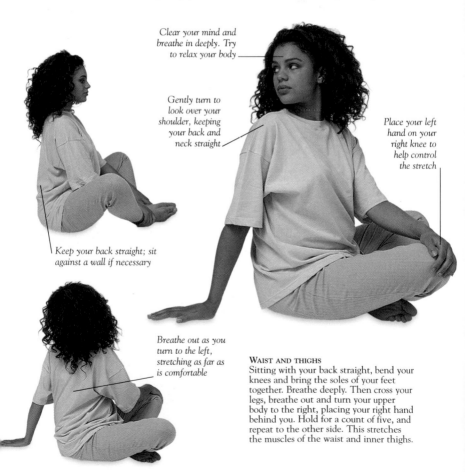

Clear your mind and breathe in deeply. Try to relax your body

Gently turn to look over your shoulder, keeping your back and neck straight

Place your left hand on your right knee to help control the stretch

Keep your back straight; sit against a wall if necessary

Breathe out as you turn to the left, stretching as far as is comfortable

WAIST AND THIGHS
Sitting with your back straight, bend your knees and bring the soles of your feet together. Breathe deeply. Then cross your legs, breathe out and turn your upper body to the right, placing your right hand behind you. Hold for a count of five, and repeat to the other side. This stretches the muscles of the waist and inner thighs.

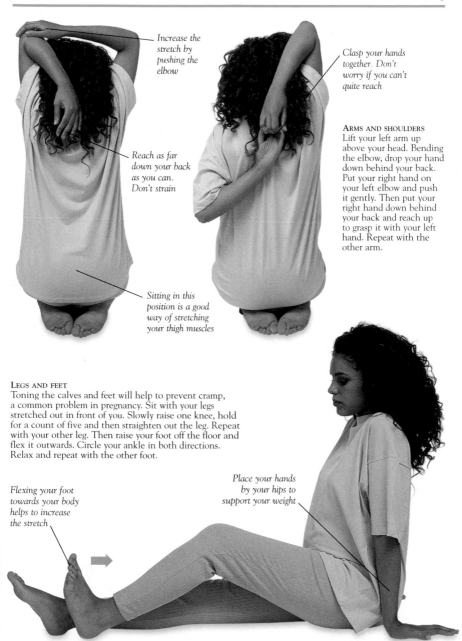

Increase the stretch by pushing the elbow

Reach as far down your back as you can. Don't strain

Sitting in this position is a good way of stretching your thigh muscles

Clasp your hands together. Don't worry if you can't quite reach

ARMS AND SHOULDERS
Lift your left arm up above your head. Bending the elbow, drop your hand down behind your back. Put your right hand on your left elbow and push it gently. Then put your right hand down behind your back and reach up to grasp it with your left hand. Repeat with the other arm.

LEGS AND FEET
Toning the calves and feet will help to prevent cramp, a common problem in pregnancy. Sit with your legs stretched out in front of you. Slowly raise one knee, hold for a count of five and then straighten out the leg. Repeat with your other leg. Then raise your foot off the floor and flex it outwards. Circle your ankle in both directions. Relax and repeat with the other foot.

Flexing your foot towards your body helps to increase the stretch

Place your hands by your hips to support your weight

Floor exercises

STRETCHING DIFFERENT PARTS of the body relieves strain and tones important muscles. Strengthening your lower back is particularly important, helping to prevent backache. By working on a firm surface and carrying out all movements smoothly, you shouldn't feel discomfort or strain. These exercises can easily be fitted into your day. Repeat each one five times to begin with, increasing slowly until you are doing 10 or 15. Don't, however, do these exercises after week 32 of pregnancy. At this late stage it's not a good idea to lie flat on your back for any length of time as the pressure of the uterus on deep veins in your pelvis may result in fainting and dizziness.

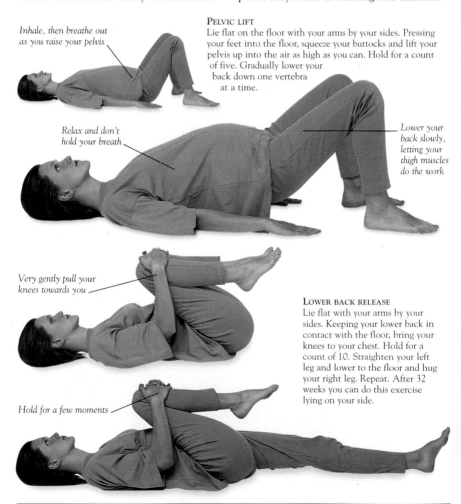

Inhale, then breathe out as you raise your pelvis

PELVIC LIFT
Lie flat on the floor with your arms by your sides. Pressing your feet into the floor, squeeze your buttocks and lift your pelvis up into the air as high as you can. Hold for a count of five. Gradually lower your back down one vertebra at a time.

Relax and don't hold your breath

Lower your back slowly, letting your thigh muscles do the work

Very gently pull your knees towards you

LOWER BACK RELEASE
Lie flat with your arms by your sides. Keeping your lower back in contact with the floor, bring your knees to your chest. Hold for a count of 10. Straighten your left leg and lower to the floor and hug your right leg. Repeat. After 32 weeks you can do this exercise lying on your side.

Hold for a few moments

SITTING EXERCISES

It's easy to neglect parts of the body like the neck or the ankles. These stretches will keep you supple and help prevent the build-up of fluid (oedema) that causes puffiness. You can do them anywhere: try them in the evening as you watch TV.

Rotate your neck slowly and carefully to avoid injury

HEAD AND NECK

Sit on the floor with your legs crossed and gently tilt your head over to one side. Lifting your chin, rotate your head back, over to the other side and down in one gentle, flowing movement. Repeat in the opposite direction. Then, keeping your head straight, turn it slowly to the right and to the left. Return to face the front.

Sitting cross-legged stretches your thigh muscles

ANKLES

Circle 5 times to the left and then to the right

Sit barefoot on the floor with your legs outstretched in front of you. Raise your right leg slightly off the ground and draw large circles in the air using only your ankles. Put your foot back on the floor and repeat with your left ankle.

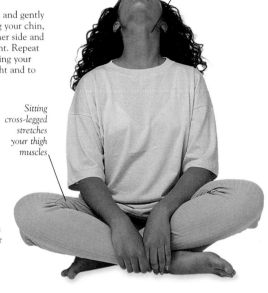

Only raise your hips a little way up from the floor

Relax your jaw. Concentrate on breathing evenly

HIP CIRCLING

Lie flat on the floor with your arms by your sides, palms down. Bend both knees and cross your feet at the ankles. Then rotate your hips clockwise, making tiny circles with your lower back on the floor. Relax and then repeat the movement in the opposite direction.

Use your arms to steady yourself

Twisting and bending

PREGNANCY HORMONES soften your ligaments in preparation for the birth; unfortunately they can also make you susceptible to strains and backache. Twisting and bending exercises help to strengthen key muscles, as well as to loosen up the pelvis in preparation for the birth. Getting down on all fours is an excellent way to ease backache, especially if you combine it with a few pelvic tilts.

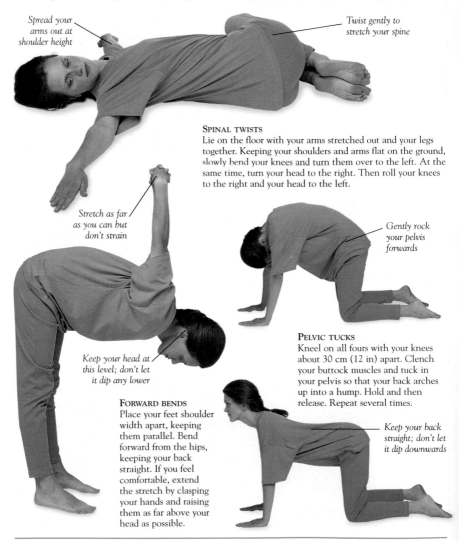

Spread your arms out at shoulder height

Twist gently to stretch your spine

SPINAL TWISTS
Lie on the floor with your arms stretched out and your legs together. Keeping your shoulders and arms flat on the ground, slowly bend your knees and turn them over to the left. At the same time, turn your head to the right. Then roll your knees to the right and your head to the left.

Stretch as far as you can but don't strain

Gently rock your pelvis forwards

Keep your head at this level; don't let it dip any lower

PELVIC TUCKS
Kneel on all fours with your knees about 30 cm (12 in) apart. Clench your buttock muscles and tuck in your pelvis so that your back arches up into a hump. Hold and then release. Repeat several times.

FORWARD BENDS
Place your feet shoulder width apart, keeping them parallel. Bend forward from the hips, keeping your back straight. If you feel comfortable, extend the stretch by clasping your hands and raising them as far above your head as possible.

Keep your back straight; don't let it dip downwards

SQUATTING

There are many benefits to be derived from doing squatting exercises. Squatting cuts off some blood from the general circulation and so gives the heart a rest. It makes your joints, especially the pelvic ones, more flexible, stretches and strengthens the thighs and back muscles and relieves back pain. Squatting is a comfortable position to relax in and is a practical position for labour and delivery (see p. 126). It may seem difficult at first but with practice it will become progressively easier.

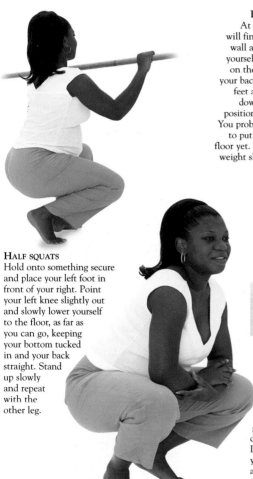

LEARNING SQUATS
At the beginning you will find it easier to use a wall and pillows to prop yourself up. Place pillows on the floor. Stand with your back against the wall, feet at hip-width. Slide down into a squatting position onto the pillows. You probably won't be able to put your heels on the floor yet. Try to keep your weight slightly forward.

HALF SQUATS
Hold onto something secure and place your left foot in front of your right. Point your left knee slightly out and slowly lower yourself to the floor, as far as you can go, keeping your bottom tucked in and your back straight. Stand up slowly and repeat with the other leg.

FULL SQUATS
Keeping your back lengthened and straight, open out your legs and squat down as low as you can. Try to get your heels on the ground with the weight evenly distributed between heels and toes. Don't worry if you have to raise your heels. If you press your elbows against your thighs, you will increase the stretch on the inner thighs and the pelvic area.

Sports activities

THERE ARE SEVERAL SPORTS that you can do as long as you take it gently and stop if you feel tired. Remember, if you are out of breath, your baby is deprived of oxygen.

WALKING

You can walk as much as you like – it's very good exercise. The main concern is that you walk under safe conditions.

SWIMMING

Swimming is an excellent form of exercise and the one sport you can continue until term. I swam two weeks before delivery with my second pregnancy, slowly and gently of course. Don't swim if the water is cold as you are more prone to cramp.

CYCLING AND DANCING

Cycling is good exercise, but stop when your abdomen gets so large that it starts to affect your centre of gravity, as you might lose your balance. As long as you're not too energetic, you can dance throughout pregnancy. It is a good way to practise pelvic tilts.

SPORTS TO AVOID

Don't go riding or skiing during pregnancy. Even if you are experienced you could fall. The risks are too great.

TAKING THE WEIGHT
As well as improving your stamina, swimming supports your weight and helps you to relax.

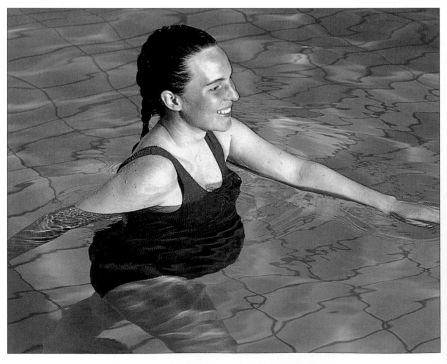

WATER EXERCISES

Swimming is wonderful exercise during pregnancy. You can improve your general fitness, while becoming more supple with the support of the water, which will help you to prepare for labour. If you don't swim, you can still do these exercises.

CYCLING MOVEMENTS
With your back to the rail, hold onto it with your arms stretched out straight. Raise your legs and make slow, exaggerated movements with your legs in the water. Keep cycling for a couple of minutes but don't become fatigued.

BODY MOVEMENTS
Facing the rail, put your feet flat against the side of the pool with your knees bent. Move your body from side to side. Stretch your legs out until they are straight out to either side, feet still flat against the side, and repeat the swaying movement.

Travelling

WHETHER SHORT OR LONG distance, travelling is unlikely to do you any harm during pregnancy, but do use your common sense. Don't risk getting tired with long, unbroken journeys, particularly on your own. Resist rough and jolting cross-country trips. Don't take travel sickness medication. Towards the end, try to stay close to home, within easy reach of your doctor.

DRIVING

You can drive until your size makes it hard to look over your shoulder, or until the wheel jams into your bump. For many women this occurs around month seven, for others there are no problems. It's illegal to stop wearing your seat belt just because you are pregnant. Some women lose their ability to make quick responses and to concentrate without a break. If you notice this happening, it is unwise to drive for any distance. If you suffer backache, make sure you have a proper support. Get out of the car at least every 160 kilometres (100 miles) and walk around to rest your joints and keep the circulation going.

TRAINS

Going by train is probably the most relaxing way to travel in pregnancy. You can stretch your legs whenever you want and there is always a toilet close by.

FLYING

Flying through time zones may be more tiring during pregnancy because of your tendency to suffer fatigue. Flying is not advisable after 36 weeks in a single pregnancy and after 32 weeks with twins or more. Airlines have different policies about flying during pregnancy and may ask for a letter from a doctor or midwife confirming fitness to fly after 28 weeks.

If you do need to fly during pregnancy, bear the following points in mind.
● Before going on a long-haul flight, ask your GP or obstetrician if you should wear anti-embolism flight socks.
● Ask the airline whether they offer any special seats or services such as early check-in for pregnant women.
● Always fasten your seatbelt below your abdomen.
● Avoid crossing your legs while seated in the plane.
● Pregnancy may increase the risk of traveller's thrombosis so all pregnant women are advised to drink plenty of water during the flight. It is not generally recommended that pregnant women take low-dose aspirin before flying.
● Walk around the cabin at least once every hour to help your circulation and carry out some foot and leg exercises. Most airlines now provide details of these, especially on long flights.

8

Looking good

In pregnancy, most women find that their skin improves and the legendary bloom appears as more blood flows under the skin, making them feel well and attractive. Exercise and a healthy diet, coupled with an awareness of the physical changes that occur in pregnancy, will contribute to your feeling happy with your changing shape and to giving you a good self-image. Taking care of your clothes, make-up and personal hygiene can also do a lot to boost morale. If you feel good, then you will probably look good too. You don't have to wear shapeless clothes; adapt your existing wardrobe for the first two trimesters.

What you wear

THE INCREASE IN THE CIRCULATION of blood throughout your body will cause you to sweat more and your vaginal secretions will also increase. It is therefore advisable to bathe daily (but never to douche) and to wear, whenever possible, lightweight natural fibres which won't irritate your skin or cause you to feel hot and restricted. Even in cold weather you will be astonished at how warm you feel, so wear fewer and lighter clothes than usual for your own comfort.

Being pregnant is nothing to be ashamed of, and fashion designers have increasingly been producing maternity clothes that accentuate your bump attractively, using fashionable colours and flattering and comfortable fabrics. These can be worn right through your pregnancy to the birth, and beyond. Bear in mind, however, that your bust size will increase so figure-hugging tops may no longer fit comfortably. Also, avoid any garments

that have a tight waistband or belt or fit closely around the thighs or crotch. Most women find that up to the fifth or sixth month they can get away with wearing their ordinary clothes, sometimes with a safety pin or a piece of velcro to help the waistbands meet. Any garments with a drawstring or an elasticated waist can be adapted as your abdomen swells.

It's a wonderful boost to your morale to invest in one or two really smart or glamorous outfits. So that you have several months to enjoy them, don't wait until your pregnancy is too advanced before going out shopping. Remember that you don't have to buy maternity clothes. From the standard dress racks you should be able to find fashionable clothes to wear.

TAKE PRIDE IN YOUR APPEARANCE
Your pregnant shape is something to be proud of and for you to enjoy. See your swelling body as something beautiful, and don't ever worry about it.

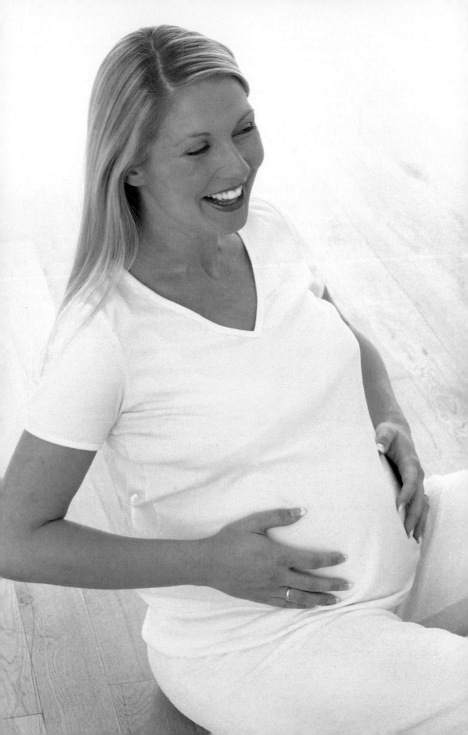

GATHERING YOUR WARDROBE

● Comfort is the watchword in pregnancy. Try to stay one step ahead of your growing size by buying clothes that are slightly too big so that you always have something to wear.

● Look in the racks of maternity clothes for ideas and make a note of the way they allow for expansion with elasticated inserts and Velcro strips, for example. You can use the same techniques to adapt your existing wardrobe.

● Front hems on maternity dresses tend to be 2.5 cm (1 in) longer than usual, so if you make your own or buy a non-maternity dress, check you have the extra fabric in the hem.

● See if there is anything in your partner's wardrobe that you might borrow, for example a sweater or a shirt.

● Replace elastic in a waistband with a drawstring.

● Loose-fitting jackets, shawls, fleeces and A-line coats are the best cover-ups.

● Choose natural fabrics such as cotton, wool or silk, which are much more comfortable than synthetics, particularly in hot weather.

● Wear layers for comfort – a long shirt over a T-shirt, for example – so that if you get too hot you can easily remove the top layer.

● Big prints and wide stripes tend to make you look larger, whereas plain colours are more subtle.

● Stretch fabrics are comfortable, but avoid clingy materials.

● For a special occasion or if you need to look smart for work, look for drop-waisted dresses or suits with long-line jackets.

● To cut the cost when buying a special outfit, visit shops that specialize in nearly-new maternity clothes.

● On the beach wear a muu-muu or sarong, or just a large T-shirt. Maternity swimwear is now readily available in department stores, and is generally both comfortable and stylish.

● A layered skirt with an elasticated or drawstring waistline can be worn under the armpits as a sundress, then pulled down and worn with a pretty top to make a versatile summer outfit.

Stylish close-fitting tops flatter your curves

CLOTHES FOR PREGNANCY
You don't need to buy a whole new wardrobe. A few special items supplemented with borrowed clothes will see you through.

A skirt with a stretchy waistband looks good and feels comfortable

Footwear

Whenever you can, go barefoot. Cotton or wool socks are often the most comfortable footwear, but tights are fine provided that they are large and stretchy enough, do not have a tight waistband, and the feet leave enough room for your toes to move freely. If you can tolerate wearing the waistband under the bump, ordinary tights will be comfortable throughout pregnancy but during the third trimester you may need special maternity tights. Don't wear garters, stockings, or knee-high socks with elastic tops because these tend to make the blood stagnate in your legs.

Your feet and back are going to take quite a strain as you get heavier and your ligaments will soften and stretch. So, for the sake of foot comfort and posture, take care when choosing shoes. It is best to avoid high heels altogether as it is difficult to stand and walk well in them. In addition they can make you unstable.

Most of the time, at least, wear low-heeled shoes that are soft and comfortable. If your feet swell, tight shoes may cut into your feet, but loose-fitting shoes can cause you to slip. Therefore, for casual wear, trainers are excellent, though the laces may be difficult to tie later in pregnancy. For summer, wear adjustable sports sandals or canvas shoes that give without pinching and allow your feet to swell freely.

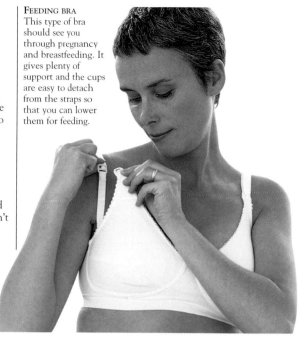

FEEDING BRA
This type of bra should see you through pregnancy and breastfeeding. It gives plenty of support and the cups are easy to detach from the straps so that you can lower them for feeding.

Bras

You should always wear a bra in pregnancy because your breasts are becoming progressively larger and heavier, putting a strain on the supporting, non-elastic tissues. If you don't lift some of the weight from these ligaments, they will stretch and your breasts will sag permanently. From the time your breasts start to get bigger, around weeks 6–8, wear a bra with a deep enough band under the cups, wide, comfortable straps and an adjustable fastening. If necessary, buy a bigger size as your breasts enlarge. If your breasts get very heavy, you may want to wear a lightweight bra at night.

If you are planning to breastfeed, by about week 36 you should buy a special bra that will allow you to feed your baby easily. Babycare shops and department stores have a wide range of styles and sizes, but if you are an unusual shape or have a narrow or wide back, see an experienced corsetier or contact one of the childbirth organizations (see p. 154). You will be wearing this bra night and day for at least six weeks (buy at least two), so it needs to feel comfortable, like a second skin. You can buy some washable or disposable breast pads now in readiness.

Skin and hair care

THERE ARE GOOD REASONS for the bloom that is said to appear on a woman's skin in pregnancy. The high level of hormones in your blood (see p. 56) affects your skin, plumping it out, giving your face a smooth, velvety appearance. Added to this, your skin acquires a rosy glow because there's more blood circulating around your body. Most women's skins improve noticeably – a dry skin becoming more supple, an oily one less shiny, and any tendency to spots disappearing – but the opposite can happen and you may have to adapt your whole beauty routine.

Your face may become plumper, which tends to smooth out lines and wrinkles, making you look younger and healthier or, conversely, even chubbier than before. You may find that your skin itches more in pregnancy, particularly over your distended stomach. Rub any kind of oil into the skin. The oil itself may not make the difference, but the massage will certainly stimulate your blood vessels and ease the irritation.

If you have put on a lot of weight, especially on your thighs, your skin may chafe. Bathe frequently, dust the area with cornflour or talcum powder and keep it dry and cool. Wear cotton and avoid nylon tights. Calamine lotion is also soothing but the only real prevention is to cut down on your weight gain.

GENERAL SKIN CARE

● Use soap as infrequently as possible on your face and body.
● Keep hand cream and lipsalve with you to use whenever necessary.
● If you wear make-up, don't stop now; make-up is good for your skin. It slows down the water loss from the skin, helping to rehydrate it.
● Use a bath oil in your bath water. It will leave a film of lubricating oil on your skin, helping to prevent water loss.

CHLOASMA

Any areas of skin that are already pigmented, such as birthmarks, moles and freckles, can darken, especially in olive-skinned brunettes. Sunlight will intensify this so keep covered up or use a sun block. Occasionally brown patches (chloasma or the mask of pregnancy) appear on the face and neck. They are caused by the pregnancy hormones (see p. 56) and are often noticed in women who take the contraceptive pill. Chloasma may be aggravated by a reaction to perfume, so test what you use. Don't try to bleach the marks out: cover them with a blemish stick, topped with a thin layer of foundation. They will go within three months of delivery. Chloasma can be brought on by sunlight and it will get worse if exposed to the sun. If you can't avoid going out in the sun, use a strong sun block. Black women may develop patches of white skin on the face and neck. These too disappear after delivery.

SPIDER VEINS

These are broken blood vessels which resemble little red spiders. They appear on the face, particularly on the cheeks. They occur when a blood vessel dilates and tiny vessels grow from this central area. They are most noticeable in fair women but will have gone within two months of delivery.

HAIR CARE

Some women notice a difference in their hair during pregnancy (see p. 63). It is a good idea to have a hairstyle that is easy to care for. You can wash your hair as often as you like, but if you notice a change in your hair, use the correct shampoo for your new hair condition. Wash your hair in the shower or use the shower attachment when you take a bath so you don't put any strain on your back.

MAKE-UP CAMOUFLAGE TRICKS

If you wear make-up, a low-key, natural look is always flattering and makes the most of a fresh complexion. A style with startling details and bright colours won't do this. Pick a foundation tone a shade paler than the skin on your neck and a translucent powder. Stay away from pink blusher shades: those in the apricot range are more natural. With your eye make-up, avoid hard colours – they will compete with the sparkle in your eyes – choose soft sludgy colours instead. A natural shade of lipstick will complete the effect. There are always ways to camouflage any bad points, or at least to minimize their effects.

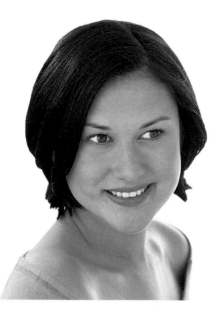

Wrinkles

If your skin becomes drier than usual, fine lines, wrinkles and crowsfeet will look more obvious. Heavy foundations will accentuate them, so choose the finest texture foundation you can get, and use a fine, translucent powder.

High colour

Increased blood supply can give you a permanently flushed look. To reduce this slightly, apply a matt beige foundation containing quite a lot of pigment but with no hint of pink in it. With your fingertips, stipple some onto the area of the cheeks where it's needed. Allow it to dry and then apply a thin layer of your usual foundation on top and finish with a colourless powder. This method is also good for concealing spider veins or any other red veins on the cheeks that become prominent.

Extra-greasy skin

For greasy patches of skin, use a water-based moisturizer and oil-free foundation with translucent powder.

Extra-dry skin

To deal with dry patches of skin, first apply a thin lotion that's absorbed by the skin within seconds, and on top apply a thicker kind that acts as a barrier to water loss. Covering the skin with a fine layer of suitable make-up also helps to slows down water loss. However, if your face is flaking, you won't be able to camouflage it, so abandon all make-up and moisturize your skin thoroughly for a few days. Consult your doctor if the flakiness is accompanied by redness.

Puffiness

It is most noticeable under the chin but can be camouflaged by shading a little brown blusher beneath the jaw-bone and either side of the neck. Apply blusher at the temples to draw attention to your eyes.

Dark circles

Apply a thin layer of foundation. When dry, stipple over the dark areas with an under-eye cover-up cream. Leave for a couple of minutes to set, then cover with another thin layer of foundation, blending carefully. Dust with colourless powder.

Acne

If you normally suffer from pimples or blackheads, you may find that they disappear. The fluctuation of hormones may, conversely, cause you to develop acne on the face or back for the first time. This is different from ordinary acne, so don't treat it with the usual proprietary preparations. Talk to your doctor if you are worried – it will usually have vanished by the second trimester.

To mask unsightly acne, stipple concealer or a little extra foundation over the area with your fingers. Finish with foundation and then dust with colourless powder.

Never squeeze a spot; this will spread germs into the deeper layers of the skin.

9

Rest and relaxation

During the first three months of pregnancy you are likely to feel surprisingly tired because, although your baby is still small, your body is having to cope with dramatic changes in hormone levels. By the second trimester, however, your body will have adjusted to these and it is quite common to feel full of energy rather than tired. It's in the last trimester, particularly the six weeks before your baby is born, that you once again feel quite exhausted and find that you need an additional two to four hours rest out of every 24. If it is difficult or impossible to arrange a routine break during the day, just take whatever chances you get to rest or relax. If possible, do this lying down, even if you don't go to sleep. And, any time you are sitting down, put your feet up if you can. If you ever feel extremely tired, don't try to battle on, give in.

Sleep

DURING PREGNANCY it is essential to get an adequate amount of sleep, and you should always aim for at least eight hours a night. Paradoxically, though, however tired and even exhausted you feel at times, you may find you suffer from insomnia. When I was pregnant with my first baby, I well remember sitting out the early hours of dawn wondering why my fatigue didn't let me sleep. I didn't know the reason for my wakefulness then, but theories now advanced suggest that a mother's wakefulness is due to the ever-present metabolism of her baby.

The baby is growing and developing all the time in the womb, around the clock, so its metabolism doesn't slow down when evening comes – its engine keeps running at top speed. This means that the mother's body has constantly to fuel her baby with food and oxygen, day and night, and her metabolism isn't allowed to slow down either. This is often reflected in her inability to sleep.
Don't fight sleeplessness and become resentful – it will only make your insomnia worse – and don't take any sleeping pills without consulting your doctor. If you can't get to sleep or keep waking

throughout the night and become increasingly restless lying in bed, try some of the following tips:

• Take the traditional remedy of a hot, milky drink before bedtime; this helps you to relax and wind down.

• Try having a warm bath before going to bed. This soothes both mind and body, making you feel sleepy and calm as well as relaxing your muscles. For many women it acts like a knockout. Be careful, however, not to have too hot a bath before you go to bed as it may stimulate rather than relax you.

• Add aromatherapy preparations to your bath water: floral essences such as lavender, rose, geranium and chamomile are best.

• Most pregnant women seem to need to spread themselves out when they sleep. If your bed is small it might be a good idea to invest in a larger one with a good supporting mattress fairly early in your pregnancy. A larger bed will also make it easier to achieve a comfortable position, propped up with several pillows, when you come to breastfeed.

• Avoid lying on your back (see p. 106). Sleep on one side instead, in a position that you find comfortable. Get hold of some extra pillows or soft cushions and experiment with using them to make yourself more at ease. For example, when lying on your side, you might want one pillow under your bump and another between your knees and thighs (see pp. 106–107).

• Even if you have difficulty getting straight off to sleep,

start going to bed earlier – you can read a good book, which will help you to relax, or do some specific relaxation exercises (see p. 103). Practise your deep breathing and concentrate on the new life inside you. Don't think of yourself as being lazy, just make sure that you get as many hours rest as you need.

• If you wake during the night, don't lie in bed fretting, get up and do something that you've been persistently putting off, or do some other useful task that could save you time next day. Make a cup of mild herb tea, such as rosehip, chamomile or peppermint, as these may help you settle to sleep again.

• Listen to some relaxing music, either on headphones in bed, or in another room.

• Make sure you don't become too hot during the night. Remember that during pregnancy your circulation increases, which can make you feel warmer. Keep your room well ventilated with the window and door open and, if necessary, change heavy duvets or blankets for lighter bedcovers.

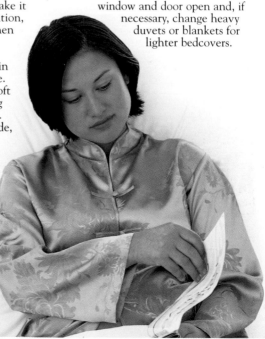

WHEN SLEEP IS DIFFICULT
Reading a book or magazine will help you to relax. Make sure you are comfortable with your back supported by pillows.

Learning how to relax

IMPATIENCE, IRRITABILITY, an inability
to concentrate and a loss of interest in sex
are all signs of fatigue. Adequate rest can
cure all of them. You can't always expect
to get sufficient sleep at night, so you need
to be alert to the possibilities of napping,
or simply relaxing with your feet up,
whenever the opportunity arises during
the day. Long naps are not essential: five
or ten minutes with your eyes closed and
your feet up can be sufficiently refreshing.
Something you'll never regret is learning
a relaxation technique, which, once
ou're accustomed to using it, can
recharge your batteries in a few minutes.
If you want to control your body so that
you can relax within 30 seconds, you
might like to practise this method of
instant relaxation or imagery training.

1 Arrange yourself comfortably.
2 Take a deep breath, hold for five seconds.
  Count to five slowly, then breathe out.
3 Tell all your muscles to relax.
4 Repeat this sequence two or three times
  until you're relaxed.
5 Imagine the most pleasant thought you
  can. A pleasant scene is ideal (see
  opposite). This helps you to use your
  imagination and to break down your
  mental blocks so that you can get more
  in touch with your body and learn to
  control it, which will be so useful
  during labour and birth.

DAYTIME REST
It is important to get enough rest, especially in the
last trimester. If you find it difficult to sleep at night
you should relax or have a catnap during the day.

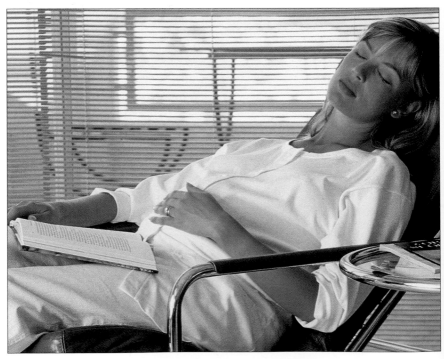

RELAXATION TECHNIQUES

PHYSICAL RELAXATION

This method involves giving orders in sequence to parts of your body to release the tension there. This is best learnt through tensing and then letting go. You will feel the difference in labour, when you should be able to relax most of the muscles in your body and let the uterus contract without the rest of your body tensing. Your partner can help you by touching you where he can see you are tensing up; you can respond to his touch by letting go.

It is best to practise this drill twice a day for 15–20 minutes if you can. Practise just before meals or an hour or more after eating.

1 Find a comfortable position lying on your back or propped up with cushions.
2 Close your eyes.
3 Think about your right hand; tense it for a moment, let it go, palm upward.
4 Tell your hand to feel heavy and warm, press your elbow into the floor or cushions, let it go.
5 Now work up through the right side of your body, through the forearm, the upper arm, into the shoulder. Raise your shoulder, let it go.
6 Repeat on the upper left side of your body. Your hands, arms and shoulders will feel heavy and warm.
7 Roll your knees outwards, relaxing your hips, and press your lower back gently into the floor or cushions. Release and let the relaxation flow into your abdomen and your chest. Tell the muscles to feel heavy and warm.
8 Your breathing should start to slow down. If it doesn't, slow it down by counting to two between each breath.
9 Now relax your neck and jaw. With your lips together, drop your jaw with your tongue on the bottom of your mouth and your cheeks loose.
10 Pay special attention to the muscles around your eyes and in your forehead; smooth away any frowns.

MENTAL RELAXATION

Once you have mastered the technique of muscle relaxation you can try relaxing your mind in this way.

1 Try clearing your mind of any stressful thoughts, anxiety or worry by breathing in and out slowly and regularly and concentrating all your attention on your breathing actions, even saying to yourself very slowly "breathe in, hold, breathe out".
2 Let pleasant thoughts flow through your head and freely associate.
3 If any worrying thought recurs, prevent it from doing so by saying "no" under your breath or return to concentrating on your deep breathing.
4 With your eyes closed, imagine a tranquil scene such as a clear, blue sky or calm, blue sea. Try to visualize something pleasant and blue because this has been found to be a particularly relaxing colour.
5 Think fairly hard about your breathing and become aware of it. Feel how it is slow and natural. Concentrate on each breath as you inhale and exhale. Listen to your breathing.
6 You should be feeling calm and restful by now – it might be helpful to repeat a soothing word or mantra such as love, peace or calm, or you may prefer a word with less symbolism such as breath, earth or laugh. Think of a word or even a calming sound like "aagh" while you are breathing out.
7 Remind yourself to keep the muscles of your face, eyes and forehead relaxed and tell your forehead to feel cool.

It might help you to settle into your relaxation method if you adopt a starting routine. For example, if you repeat a mantra or drop your shoulders this can be the signal to the rest of your body to begin. Whenever you practise a relaxation method, make sure that you are breathing deeply, in the most controlled way (see p. 104).

Breathing techniques

PART OF YOUR TIME in antenatal classes will be spent learning how to relax and master the various breathing techniques. It's important to learn different types of breathing; you can use each one at different times during labour to help you to relax, conserve energy, control your body and pain, to calm you and stop you being afraid. Realizing that you can exert some control over your body through breathing techniques will give you more confidence during labour. Here are three basic levels that will help you. Practise them with your partner, or whoever will be with you at the birth, so you can both learn the techniques to help you through labour.

DEEP BREATHING

When you breathe in you should feel the lowermost part of your lungs fill with air and your lower ribcage expand outwards and upwards. Drop your shoulders. If someone places their hands on your lower back, you should be able to move their hands with your inhalation. It feels like the end of a sigh and is followed by a slow, deep exhalation. This produces a calming influence and is ideal for the beginning and end of contractions.

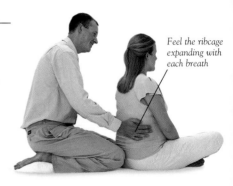

Feel the ribcage expanding with each breath

LIGHT BREATHING

Aerate only the upper part of your lungs so that the top part of your chest and your shoulder blades lift and expand. Your partner can feel this if she places her hands on your shoulder blades. Your breaths should be fast and short with your lips slightly apart. Draw the breath in through your throat. After 10 or so light breaths you may need to take a deep breath – do so. This level of breathing is useful when used in labour at the height of a contraction.

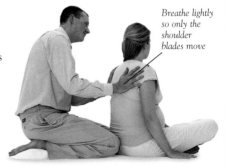

Breathe lightly so only the shoulder blades move

FEATHERLIGHT BREATHING

The method I found most useful was panting. This is taking shallow breaths and resembles what you see and hear when a dog pants. Think of this as "pant, pant, blow". One of the times when you will be asked to pant is during transition to stop you bearing down before the cervix is fully dilated (see p. 124). When you're taking short, rapid, shallow breaths, the diaphragm is contracting and relaxing quickly and this prevents you from making a downward, concerted push. It's also useful to pant right through a painful contraction as you won't feel out of breath at the end. To stop yourself overbreathing, or hyperventilating, pant 10–15 times and then hold your breath for a count of five.

MASSAGE

Physical contact is a source of comfort and solace at any time, but especially during pregnancy. Massage can be used as a means of relaxing you, and it also brings you and your partner close together. It's very useful during the first stages of labour, not only for relieving back pain but also for helping to reassure and soothe you.

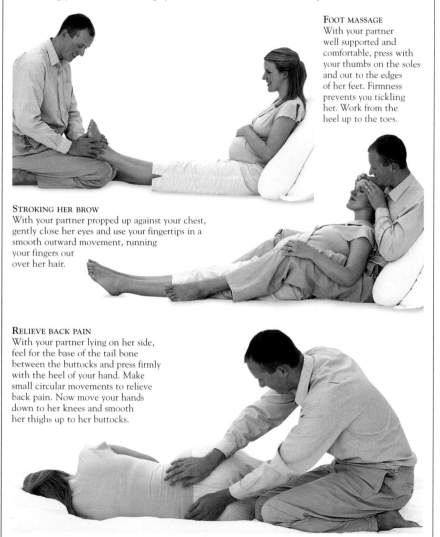

FOOT MASSAGE
With your partner well supported and comfortable, press with your thumbs on the soles and out to the edges of her feet. Firmness prevents you tickling her. Work from the heel up to the toes.

STROKING HER BROW
With your partner propped up against your chest, gently close her eyes and use your fingertips in a smooth outward movement, running your fingers out over her hair.

RELIEVE BACK PAIN
With your partner lying on her side, feel for the base of the tail bone between the buttocks and press firmly with the heel of your hand. Make small circular movements to relieve back pain. Now move your hands down to her knees and smooth her thighs up to her buttocks.

Comfortable positions

AS YOUR ABDOMEN gets larger, sitting or lying in your usual positions can become uncomfortable. If you lie flat on your back for any length of time, especially in later pregnancy, the baby's weight presses down on major blood vessels running up your

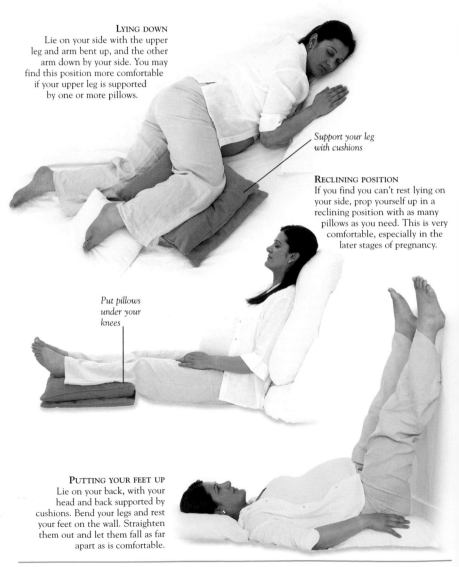

LYING DOWN
Lie on your side with the upper leg and arm bent up, and the other arm down by your side. You may find this position more comfortable if your upper leg is supported by one or more pillows.

Support your leg with cushions

RECLINING POSITION
If you find you can't rest lying on your side, prop yourself up in a reclining position with as many pillows as you need. This is very comfortable, especially in the later stages of pregnancy.

Put pillows under your knees

PUTTING YOUR FEET UP
Lie on your back, with your head and back supported by cushions. Bend your legs and rest your feet on the wall. Straighten them out and let them fall as far apart as is comfortable.

back. This can make you uncomfortable and dizzy as your blood pressure drops and it can aggravate haemorrhoids. For these reasons, it's not advisable to sleep, rest or exercise on your back. Carefully arranged pillows and floor cushions help, but don't lie with too many pillows under your head or your spine will be too curved. When sitting, don't cross your legs or bend them tightly as this may aggravate varicose veins. Try the positions below and always be aware of maintaining good posture.

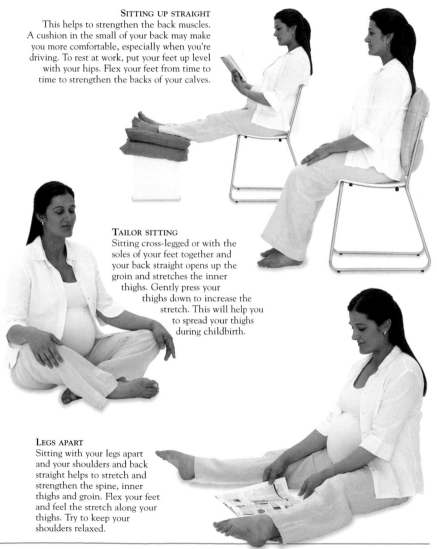

SITTING UP STRAIGHT
This helps to strengthen the back muscles. A cushion in the small of your back may make you more comfortable, especially when you're driving. To rest at work, put your feet up level with your hips. Flex your feet from time to time to strengthen the backs of your calves.

TAILOR SITTING
Sitting cross-legged or with the soles of your feet together and your back straight opens up the groin and stretches the inner thighs. Gently press your thighs down to increase the stretch. This will help you to spread your thighs during childbirth.

LEGS APART
Sitting with your legs apart and your shoulders and back straight helps to stretch and strengthen the spine, inner thighs and groin. Flex your feet and feel the stretch along your thighs. Try to keep your shoulders relaxed.

10

Preparing for the birth

By the 36th week of your pregnancy, you should have given up work and be slowing down your social and domestic routines. You may feel frustrated and bored or you may welcome the rest from your work and the travel to and fro or feel energized and want to spring-clean the house from top to bottom. This is the time to check that everything is ready for the new arrival – the room, the clothing, the equipment – and to prepare yourself, your partner and your other children for the birth.

Organizing your home

THERE ARE MANY THINGS you can do to prepare yourself and the household to cover your day-to-day routine and to make life easier for you after the baby is born.

● If you haven't already got one, invest in a tumble drier. It will make the extra work so much easier, especially if you choose terry nappies.

● Start to neglect certain parts of your domestic life. Allow the non-essentials to slide and don't worry about them.

● Stop doing any housework that involves hard physical effort.

● Make sure that your family realizes that you can't dash around as you used to. Get others to help with errands.

● Try not to worry about things that don't matter. The highest priority is the baby that is growing inside you. Try to judge your pace and don't overdo anything.

● Sound out a reliable neighbour who will help in emergencies.

● If you have a freezer, stock it with staple foods that freeze well, such as bread, butter, soups, casseroles and vegetables.

● Stock up your food cupboard with tins and dried foods and buy in basic essentials such as soap powder, toilet rolls and disposable nappies.

GETTING THE BABY'S ROOM READY

If you have enough space, you can give the baby a separate room and make it into a nursery, but this isn't absolutely necessary – your baby's space can be a corner of a larger room. Even if you have planned a nursery, you'll probably find you hardly use it in the early weeks after

PREPARING THE NURSERY
Once you have the essential items like a cot and bedding, you can enjoy decorating the nursery – you'll have little time once your baby is born.

delivery. You'll find it much more convenient to have your baby with you in your bedroom, particularly at night, and close by you in his carrycot or crib the rest of the time. After these early weeks, it is ideal to have a room that is specially designed and equipped for all your baby's routines, such as feeding, bathing, changing, dressing and playing.

There is no need to go to a lot of expense. Your baby will grow quickly and soon require different things, so there is little point in investing a great deal of money in baby equipment. Before long you'll be adapting the nursery to a toddler's bedroom. Most of the equipment can be purchased second-hand. Look around in local papers and shop windows or at your baby clinic.

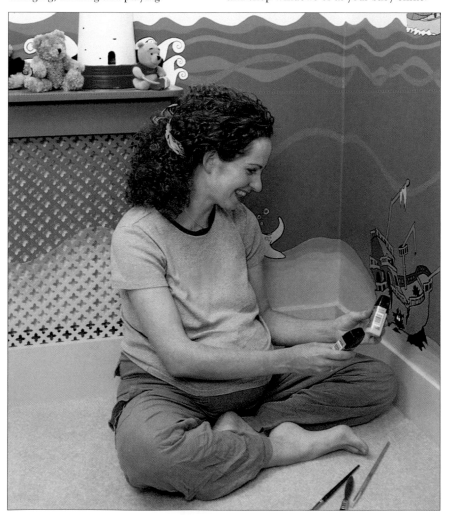

What you need for your baby

IT'S HELPFUL to start thinking about what you need for your baby quite early in your pregnancy, particularly if you're planning any structural changes to your home.

NURSERY EQUIPMENT

● Crib and cot – a crib is a luxury for the first few months. Your baby can just as easily sleep in a Moses basket or in a carrycot. A tiny baby can sleep in a full-size cot provided you do not impede air circulation with a cot bumper and you lie him down "feet to foot" – so that his feet are touching the foot of the cot and he cannot wriggle down under the blankets.

● Moses basket – this can be useful for up to six months depending on the size and vigour of your baby. It can be used as an alternative crib.

● A rear-facing baby car seat with carry handles that can be secured to the front or back seat of the car.

● For the crib or cot, choose a firm, flat mattress with a waterproof cover. Babies should never have pillows as they might suffocate in the fabric covers.

● Towelling fitted sheets or flannelette for warmth – at least 4–5.

● Only use cotton cellular blankets; wool may make him too hot. Duvets should not be used for babies under 12 months.

ESSENTIAL BABY CLOTHING

● 6 stretch suits – you may be showered with tiny clothes for the baby. The first size only lasts about 6 weeks but you will need several because of frequent soiling.

● 2 nightdresses – these make nappy changing easy.

● 4 vests – envelope necks are best.

● 2 cardigans or jumpers – avoid lacy patterns which are impractical as they catch around little fingers.

● 2 pairs cotton socks or bootees.

● 1 bonnet.

● Muslin squares for catching possets and protecting your clothing during burping sessions. They can also be stretched across the cot under the baby's head to catch any posset and protect the sheet.

● Nappies – you can opt for reusable nappies or disposables, or a combination of the two. Studies have shown that when nappies, nappy cleansing solution and electricity for the washing machine are added up, disposables are not that much more expensive. You must decide. Use disposables for the first few weeks to give yourself a break from the washing. If you use terry nappies, buy at least two dozen good-quality nappies, either shaped nappies with Velcro fastenings or terry towelling squares with separate nappy pins. You will also need two plastic buckets with lids, and cleansing solution.

● Nappy liners – disposable liners are useful inside terry nappies as they can contain stools and thus reduce staining.

● At least six pairs of plastic pants if you are using terry nappies. They quickly become brittle and crack. So buy the best quality and try to wash them by hand.

● Baby bath – this is useful as it means you can bath your baby in the warmest place, not necessarily in the bathroom. It's best to wait till your baby is about four months old before using the big bath.

● Plastic changing mat.

● Two soft new towels for the baby's use – your own towels will feel like sandpaper against the baby's perfect skin.

● Baby bath solution or baby soap.

● Natural sponge or soft facecloths.

● Cotton wool.

● Vaseline, cleansing lotion, toilet rolls or baby wipes for changing time.

● Arachis oil or olive oil for flaky skin.

● Blunt-ended scissors.

● A changing bag – it unfolds to reveal a waterproof area for changing the baby and has pockets all around that hold nappies, change of clothes, cleansing lotion and nappy pins. It can then be rolled up and

slung over your shoulder after the change.
● Pram or pushchair – you will have to do a lot of research here to decide on your needs. If you have a car and drive everywhere, a pram with collapsible frame is perfect. If you travel on public transport, a pushchair that collapses easily and adjusts to the horizontal position is ideal. There are so many designs now, so shop around and ask other parents.
● Sling and back pack – the sling is for the first six months or so, depending on the weight of the baby, but a back pack for an older baby can also be useful, especially for a baby who has become accustomed to being carried around.
● Feeding equipment if you are not breastfeeding, or if you express milk for someone else to feed to your baby.

Nursery floor plan
Work out your own requirements by drawing up a floor plan of your baby's room to scale. Make sure that you take account of the position of doors, windows, radiators, and electric sockets and switches.

● A bouncing cradle – in this reclining seat the baby can be partly propped up and can see you moving around the room.

Arranging a nursery

See that all the surfaces in the nursery are hygienic and easy to wipe clean. Make sure that there is plenty of storage space, especially around the changing area. Open shelves for storage mean that it is easy to reach your baby's belongings, but floor-level cupboards will need baby locks later on when your baby becomes more mobile and inquisitive.

Fit a washable floor covering and a dimmer switch for night feeds. Heat control is also important; the temperature should be constant at around 18–20°C (65–68°F), so your baby is neither too hot nor too cold. For your comfort you'll need a low feeding chair and a table. It may be a bit of a luxury, but if it's possible, install a small sink with running water in the corner of the room.

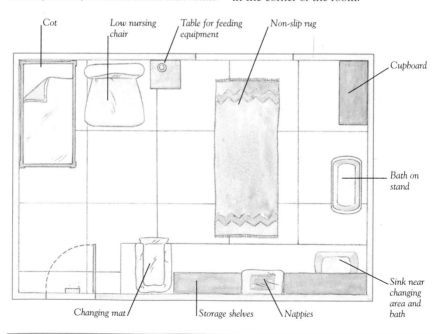

Cot
Low nursing chair
Table for feeding equipment
Non-slip rug
Cupboard
Bath on stand
Sink near changing area and bath
Changing mat
Storage shelves
Nappies

Getting ready for the birth

THE HOSPITAL OR YOUR MIDWIFE will give you a list of the items you will need for the birth. If you are having your baby at home, you will need to prepare a room for the birth.

PREPARING FOR A HOME BIRTH

There are some useful ways you can make your home birth comfortable for yourself and convenient for the midwife.
● Make sure your bed is firm so that you have something to push against and you can avoid getting a puddle of amniotic fluid under your hips. If necessary, put a board under the mattress. You may decide

not to use the bed but have it ready so that all your options are open.
● The most convenient way to make the bed is as follows. Make it up with fresh sheets. Put on a plastic sheet (an old shower curtain will do) and cover with clean old linens. In this way the old sheets and plastic can be taken off after the birth, leaving you in a freshly made bed.
● Provide polythene sheeting to protect furniture and flooring in the room in which you are going to give birth.
● Prepare a work area, such as a table top or a dressing-table, that is within easy reach of the bed for supplies.
● The maternity pack provided by the

EQUIPMENT FOR A HOME BIRTH

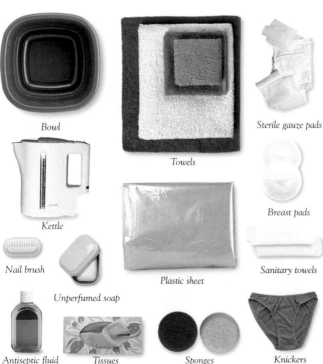

Bowl

Towels

Sterile gauze pads

Kettle

Breast pads

Nail brush

Plastic sheet

Sanitary towels

Unperfumed soap

Antiseptic fluid

Tissues

Sponges

Knickers

EXTRA ITEMS
As well as the items shown and the equipment provided by your midwife, you may also like to have the following items to hand:
● hot-water bottle for comfort during labour and for soothing afterpains
● nourishing, easily digested snacks and drinks
● hand mirror to help you see the birth
● camera and plenty of film
● presents for siblings
● a supply of paper knickers can also be very useful.

AIDS FOR LABOUR

For hospital delivery your partner or birth assistant will also need to pack a small bag with aids for the labour. Prepare and take with you a bag containing:
● a small natural sponge to moisten her mouth
● Lipsalve or Vaseline to prevent her lips becoming chapped
● frozen picnic freezing pack or hot water bottle to put against her back if she has bad backache
● a vacuum flask of diluted fruit juice or water (check if the hospital allows) for her

to sip during labour
● drinks and sandwiches for yourself and enough left over for her if after delivery she's just missed a meal
● books, playing cards, scrabble, jigsaws, cassette player and tapes to occupy you both while you're waiting between contractions
● coins for the hospital phone box
● leg warmers or thick socks if she starts to shiver during the later stages (see p. 124)
● facecloth to mop her face if she becomes too hot.

midwife before the birth will contain many of the items necessary for the birth. Check with your midwife to see if she will bring a sterile sheet.
● Clear a large area if you plan to have a mobile labour. Have some freshly ironed sheets nearby in case you prefer to deliver on the floor when the time comes.
● To prepare yourself you should have a bath, or a shower to avoid infection if the waters have broken. Otherwise, wash your hands to beyond the wrists, wash your thighs 30cm (12in) down either side, wash the pubic area, all with antiseptic soap, and dry with a clean towel, sterile cloth or gauze pad.
● Have ready a clean nightdress, sanitary pads and underpants for yourself, and a cotton cellular blanket, a disposable nappy and a nightdress or stretch suit for the baby. Prepare the cot with the baby's bedding and blankets in place.

WHAT TO TAKE TO HOSPITAL

Several weeks before your baby is due, pack your hospital case with all the things you will need for your stay there. Ask the hospital if they provide a clothes list. Few hospitals provide nappies or baby clothes during your stay, though most provide bedding. You may find that your partner has to fetch and carry clean and soiled clothing during your stay, and then will have to bring in day clothes for you and

something for the baby to wear when you are discharged from hospital. Remember to set aside loose-fitting clothes. Your breasts will have increased greatly in size when the milk comes in and your abdomen won't have gone down yet.

FOR YOU

● 2–3 front-opening nightdresses
● 2–3 maternity bras (see p. 97)
● breast pads
● dressing gown
● slippers
● 4 pairs of pants
● sanitary towels – get the most absorbent you can find for the first few days until the lochia subsides
● toilet bag and contents – hair brush, 2 towels, 2 facecloths
● tissues or a soft toilet roll
● make-up, face and hand cream and shampoo
● mirror
● coins or card for the telephone

FOR THE BABY

You are likely to need:
● 1 packet newborn-size disposable nappies
● 3 vests
● 3 stretch suits or nighties
● cotton cellular blanket

Involving your other children

IF YOU HAVE A FAMILY, every member should be involved in your pregnancy. Children should be informed about what is going on and how the pregnancy is progressing, according to their age and how much information they can absorb and understand. Even a very young child will notice that your abdomen is swelling and will want to know why. Give an honest and accurate answer and let your child feel the baby kicking inside you. If your child or children are old enough, put a chart up on the wall of what happens to you and the baby in pregnancy and follow it through as your pregnancy progresses.

If you are having a home confinement you must decide whether you want your children to be involved or not. It is sensible not to restrict the child and if he follows your pregnancy through, the experience will be an enlightening one. Don't be surprised, though, if he gets bored at the time and wants to go off and play. Someone responsible must be there, besides your partner, to take care of him during the labour.

Run through everything with him, especially the fact that it is a bit painful and you are likely to call out, otherwise he may be frightened. You should also prepare

him for the birth of the placenta, which is often the bloodiest part. Warn him that you won't be able to answer his questions because you'll be busy and that if the midwife asks him to leave the room, he must do as she says and not hesitate.

If you are going into hospital, explain to your child what is going to happen and what arrangements will be

KEEPING YOUR CHILDREN INFORMED
Chart the progress of your pregnancy with your older children and involve them with it as much as possible so they understand what is happening.

made, as long as he is old enough to understand. Even if you will be in hospital for a short time, say 24 or 48 hours, you will have to make arrangements for someone to take care of your child. If you possibly can, ask someone he knows well to come and look after him in his own home so that his normal routine isn't disrupted too much and he has all his familiar objects around him. If this isn't possible and he has to be looked after in someone else's home, make sure it's somewhere with which he is familiar and where he has spent the night more than once well before the birth – you may have a long labour and so it could be 18–24 hours before your partner is able to collect him.

Make sure that your child knows exactly how long you are likely to be apart. Prepare him in other ways by pointing out small babies to him; show him pictures of his own babyhood and relate this to the coming arrival. Buy him a doll of his own so that he feels he has a baby too. It helps too if your partner increases his involvement with the child, particularly with the usual routines of bathing, feeding and storytelling.

If your child is old enough to understand, it will help if you can rehearse what is going to happen so that he becomes familiar with the future events. It is surprise that will upset him. Compile a timetable of what you will do when labour starts and go over this with him in detail so he becomes familiar with the scenario. If you rehearse the whole scheme together several times he will feel happy and secure in the knowledge that you are taking special care of him.

COUNTDOWN FOR LABOUR

Home confinement
1 Ring the midwife.
2 Ring your partner or birth assistant.
3 Contact whoever is caring for your other children and alert them.
4 Make yourself a hot drink.
5 Check that the room is ready.
6 Have a hot bath or shower.

Hospital confinement
1 Ring the hospital, then call an ambulance or taxi if you are not being driven in by your partner or a friend. Don't drive yourself.
2 Ring your partner or birth assistant.
3 Alert whoever is caring for your children that you are going in.
4 Make yourself a hot drink.
5 Collect together your handbag, coat and your packed bag.
6 Sit down and wait for your partner or the ambulance.

If someone is driving you to the hospital, you should know how to get there and how long it will take. Plot an alternative route in case the traffic is heavy or you find the road blocked for some reason. Whenever possible, choose well-made roads so that your journey will be comfortable. Find out which hospital entrance you should use, during the day and night, to get you to the ward by the most direct route. Make sure you and the driver are thoroughly familiar with all this information and, if it puts your mind at rest, do a trial run.

Signs of labour
In the week or two before you go into labour you may experience signs that something is about to happen.
1 You feel a "lightening" or engagement, when the baby's head drops into the pelvis.
2 The baby's engagement causes an increase in pressure on the bladder and you will find that you want to pass urine more frequently again.
3 Braxton Hicks contractions become more frequent and may get stronger.
4 Often vaginal secretions increase a day or so before labour starts. If it's your first baby you may have a "show" (see p. 17) as much as two weeks before labour.
5 You may notice slight weight loss in the last week.
6 Some women experience a nesting instinct, wanting to clean the house.

11

Labour and birth

This is the high point to which all your preparations during pregnancy have been leading. While it would be unrealistic to expect the birth to be pain-free, you can hope for it to be relaxed and happy. You will be pleased, despite the discomfort, if everything and everyone around you are known to you. You will be relaxed if you understand what is happening to you and are confident that you can control your body and help during the delivery. If you learn about labour and birth and practise the exercises and breathing techniques, you should feel less pain and be alert to enjoy giving birth.

Labour

LABOUR CAN BE DIVIDED into well-defined stages. There is a stage before labour begins, sometimes called pre-labour. The first labour stage is divided into two; the early phase is when you start going into labour and when contractions may be short, irregular and not too painful. This culminates in the late first stage of labour and the transition when your contractions become regular, more frequent and painful and result in full dilatation of the cervix. The second stage of labour is when you push the baby through the birth canal and it ends with the birth of your baby. Labour is not complete until you have gone through the third stage, which is delivery of the placenta (afterbirth).

PAIN IN LABOUR

Every woman feels the pain of contractions differently but in early labour they may be similar to menstrual cramps and sometimes they're confined to mild backache. The kind of labour that proceeds well into the first stage with nothing more than gradually worsening backache is often called a backache labour (see p. 124). Very often a contraction feels like a wave of discomfort across your abdomen that reaches a crescendo for a few seconds and then diminishes. At the same time you can feel a hardening and tightening of the uterine muscle, which is held at the peak of its intensity for a few seconds and then begins to relax. You have no control over your contractions – they are "involuntary" – though your state of mind during labour can have a profound effect on contractions, making them feel more or less painful.

Most women assume that contractions will get longer, more frequent and stronger in a steady pattern. This is not so and don't be disturbed if your contractions seem to vary. It is absolutely normal for a strong contraction, for example, to be followed by a weaker one that doesn't last quite as long. It is also normal for contractions to follow one another relentlessly – this is more likely if labour has been induced and is kept going with an intravenous drip (see pp. 140–141).

ONSET OF LABOUR

Most people think the onset of labour will be very clear; pains will come, contractions will start and you'll know. It often isn't clear at all. Three things might happen, though they don't necessarily mean that birth is imminent.
• The blood-tinged, gelatinous plug of mucus that has blocked the cervical canal may be dislodged during the early first stage of labour (although this can happen as much as two weeks beforehand), and always precedes rupture of the membranes. It is sometimes called the show and means that the cervix is beginning to stretch.
• Your membranes may rupture at any time up to the delivery. Leakage of the amniotic fluid varies from being a gush to a slight dribble that can be stemmed by wearing a sanitary pad. There is no pain accompanying rupture of the membranes and the flow depends on the site and size of the break and whether or not the baby's

LENGTH OF LABOUR

Labour is usually longest with a first baby, an average 12–14 hours. Thereafter labour lasts an average seven hours. In general, the lighter the contractions, the longer the labour will be. A fast labour tends to start with long, slow contractions and proceeds in the same way.

head can plug the hole. If the membranes have ruptured you should contact the midwife or the hospital immediately.
• You may feel a dull backache or, if you had Braxton Hicks contractions during the third trimester, you may mistake the early contractions of labour for stronger Braxton Hicks. Severe Braxton Hicks can be mistaken for labour, however, and this is known as a "false labour". Time these early contractions over an hour and if they get closer together and longer in duration, you're probably in labour. The intervals between contractions once it's established that you're in labour are timed from the end of one to the beginning of the next. The contractions tend to be 30–60 seconds long at first, building up gradually to 75 seconds during the most active phase of labour.

THE PRESENTATION

The presenting part of your baby is the part that will be born first. Most babies lie in a well-flexed (curled-up) position with the chin resting on the chest (near right). The way the baby presents can affect labour and birth; a posterior presentation (far right) can lead to an erratic backache labour (see p. 124). If the face is presenting, labour may be slower and the baby's features may be slightly swollen for about 24 hours.

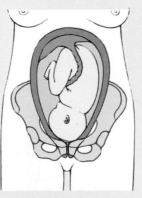

WELL-FLEXED POSITION

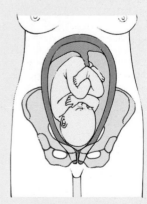

POSTERIOR PRESENTATION

ADMISSION TO HOSPITAL

When you reach the labour ward the midwife will prepare you for the birth. Your birth attendant can stay with you while she does this.

● She will consult your notes and ask you about the labour so far – whether your waters have gone, how frequently the contractions are coming and whether or not you have moved your bowels.

● She will ask you to change into the loose clothes you have brought with you to wear for the labour and birth.

INITIAL EXAMINATION

When you arrive in the maternity unit, a doctor or midwife will gently feel your abdomen so that she can establish which way the baby is facing.

● You will be examined; the midwife will palpate your abdomen to feel the baby's position, she will listen to the fetal heart-beat, take your blood pressure, pulse and temperature, and you'll be given an internal examination to see how far your cervix has dilated. She may record the fetal heart on an electronic monitor for up to 30 minutes.

● You will be asked to give a urine sample to test for protein and sugar.

● You can then have a shower or bath if you like, and make yourself comfortable in the delivery room with the help of your birth partner and the midwife. If you have any questions or you want to discuss your birthplan and make your feelings known to the staff, now is the time to remind them of your preferences.

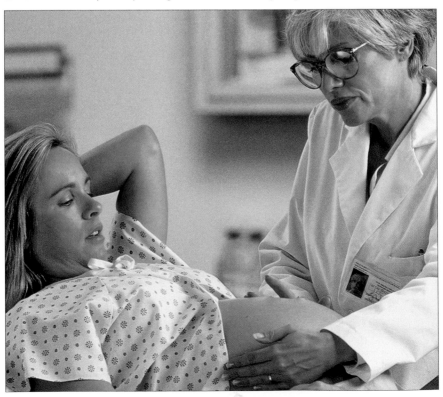

BREATHING FOR LABOUR AND BIRTH

If you have practised a relaxation technique (see p. 103) and have learnt to recognize the different types or levels of breathing, now is the time to put them into practice. Your birth assistant will be able to help you by reminding you when your breathing is too rapid or your shoulders are tense. The birth assistant can help by tapping out a rhythm or using words like "breath, breath, pant, pant, blow".

EARLY FIRST STAGE
The contractions in the early stages will probably be gentle and you should be able to breathe deeply and evenly throughout. Greet each contraction with a slow, even breath out.

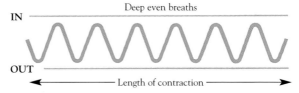

LATE FIRST STAGE
Take your opening breath out and then try to breathe above the contractions; light, short breaths that hardly seem to involve the lower parts of your body at all. Take a deep breath and relax when it is all over, to signal to yourself and those around you that the contraction is over.

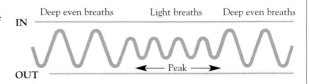

TRANSITION
If you want to push too early, try the shallowest breathing of all – panting – though without hyperventilating and starving your body of carbon dioxide. Breathe only in your mouth. If you feel dizzy, your birth assistant can cup his hands over your nose and mouth while you are breathing.

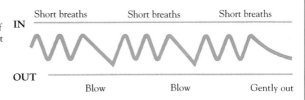

SECOND STAGE
This should be the most natural pattern of breathing for you. Take a deep breath and hold it while bearing down and letting your pelvic floor bulge outward. Let your push be long and smooth. Then repeat if the contraction is still intense; relax when it ends.

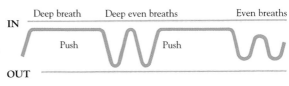

The first stage of labour

DURING THIS STAGE the cervix opens out (dilates) to allow the baby's head to pass through. Before it dilates, the cervix becomes thinned and softened and is gradually pulled up by the contracting uterine muscle. This is called effacement. The muscle of the upper segment of the uterus contracts and puts pressure on the lower segment, which in turn transmits the pull of the contractions to the cervix. As a result, once the cervix has stretched, it dilates with each contraction until the entire cervical canal is eliminated. You are then fully dilated. The degrees of dilatation of the cervix have been standardized so that it can be described

accurately and progress can be charted. If you ask the midwife how labour is progressing, she will probably respond in terms of the number of centimetres of cervical dilatation or perhaps with the number of fingers (one finger is about one centimetre).

Dilatation is normally given in one-centimetre increments up to 10 centimetres. When the cervix is said to be fully dilated it is approximately 10 centimetres in diameter. This is the completion of the first stage of labour, though in real terms the first stage often moves gradually and smoothly into the second stage without punctuation.

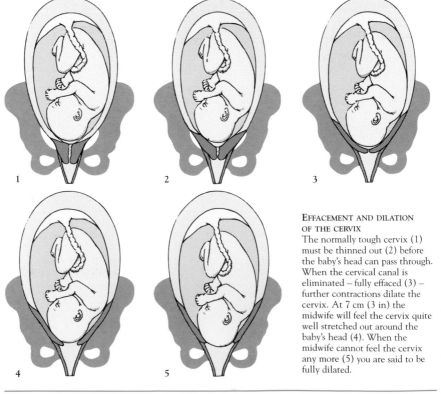

1

2

3

4

5

EFFACEMENT AND DILATION OF THE CERVIX
The normally tough cervix (1) must be thinned out (2) before the baby's head can pass through. When the cervical canal is eliminated – fully effaced (3) – further contractions dilate the cervix. At 7 cm (3 in) the midwife will feel the cervix quite well stretched out around the baby's head (4). When the midwife cannot feel the cervix any more (5) you are said to be fully dilated.

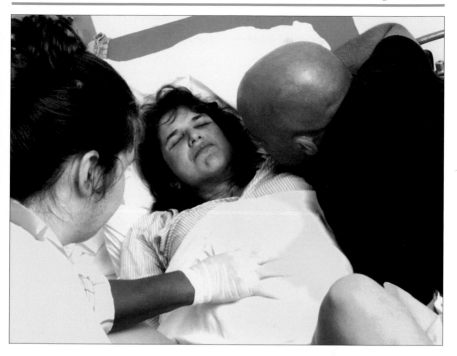

EXAMINATIONS DURING LABOUR

If you have asked for an epidural, an anaesthetist will visit you after the admission procedure. If not, you will be left with your partner or birth assistant and a nurse or midwife will be with you throughout your labour.

The fetal heart will be regularly monitored either by fetoscope, sonicaid or a machine (see p. 142). Internal examinations will be done every four hours to check progress if all is going well. Examinations may be more frequent if there are problems or if the midwife is concerned. The midwife will do this while you are sitting up or lying on your side on the bed. Let her know which position you prefer. It is more difficult for the midwife to examine you while standing.

The midwife who examines you may or may not be one of the team who has been looking after you throughout. She will let

ASSESSING PROGRESS
Your caregivers will check how far your cervix has dilated and will tell you how well you are doing.

you know that it is time to examine you and will tell you how things are progressing. Ask her, or get your partner to ask her, if you don't understand something. If you feel that your contractions are getting longer and stronger and you haven't had an internal examination for a while, then ask for one. It is quite cheering to find that your cervical dilatation has progressed between examinations.

There is not usually any problem about your companion being allowed to stay with you while you have internal examinations, but it is your choice.

You may be asked questions during an internal examination or while you are having a contraction. Concentrate on what you are doing and answer the question when the contraction is over.

POSITIONS FOR THE FIRST STAGE

There is no single "correct" position for labour; you need to experiment and find the most comfortable position for you. Move around and keep trying new positions. You can use the furniture or your partner for support if you like. Many women like to move around and when the contraction starts, take up their chosen position.

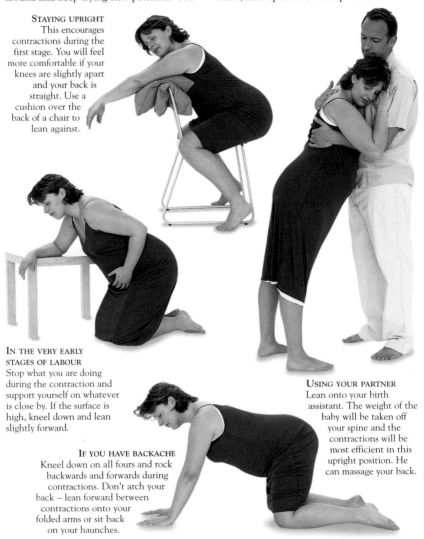

STAYING UPRIGHT
This encourages contractions during the first stage. You will feel more comfortable if your knees are slightly apart and your back is straight. Use a cushion over the back of a chair to lean against.

IN THE VERY EARLY STAGES OF LABOUR
Stop what you are doing during the contraction and support yourself on whatever is close by. If the surface is high, kneel down and lean slightly forward.

IF YOU HAVE BACKACHE
Kneel down on all fours and rock backwards and forwards during contractions. Don't arch your back – lean forward between contractions onto your folded arms or sit back on your haunches.

USING YOUR PARTNER
Lean onto your birth assistant. The weight of the baby will be taken off your spine and the contractions will be most efficient in this upright position. He can massage your back.

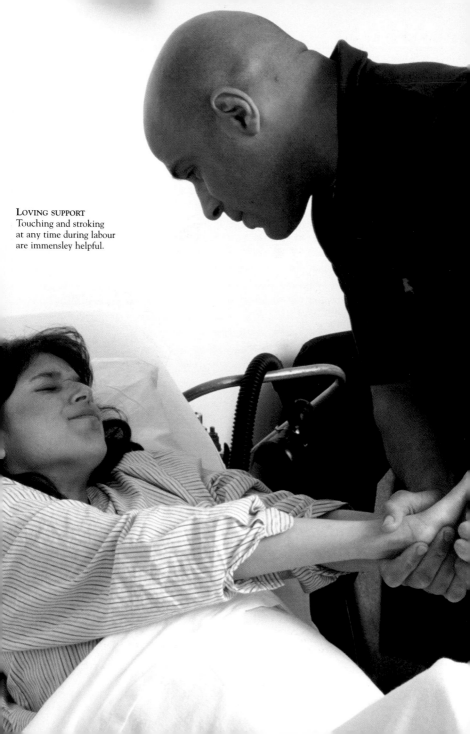

LOVING SUPPORT
Touching and stroking
at any time during labour
are immensley helpful.

THE TRANSITIONAL STAGE

This is the period from the end of the first stage of labour to the beginning of the second stage. Not all women experience it as a well-defined, distinct stage of labour, but some do and it is as well to be prepared. It rarely lasts for more than an hour, often much less, but it can be quite hard to cope with. Coming at the end of several hours in the first stage, some women become discouraged and feel that they can't go on without pain relief. There may be some shaking and shivering, which is physiological and not abnormal. Simply because of all the hormone changes that are going on you may feel some irritability and ill-temper and some women feel so nauseous that they want to vomit. Don't resist this urge because you will feel a lot better afterwards. You may feel excited and restless; every position seems uncomfortable. You may feel anxious for your own safety and for the baby's, and you may feel sleepy between contractions because most of the oxygen in your body is being taken up by the uterus and the baby, and your brain is relatively short of it.

Some women feel the urge to push during this stage but don't bear down until it is confirmed that you are fully dilated. If you feel a strong urge to push but it is too soon to do so, use the panting and blowing breathing technique (see p. 104) until the midwife tells you it is safe to start to push.

ADVICE TO BIRTH ASSISTANT

● Try to get her to relax. Refrain from asking questions and remove perspiration if she's sweating a lot.
● If she tells you not to touch her, refrain but stay near the bed. If she feels sick and wants to vomit, get a basin and encourage her to do so. Always praise her.
● If her legs start to tremble, put on her socks and hold her legs firmly.
● If you notice that she is beginning to grunt and make pushing movements, let the midwife know immediately. This is a difficult time for your partner, and you can encourage her by explaining that you think she is in transition, stage two is beginning and the baby will soon be born.
● You will know that the delivery is imminent when the midwife says that the head is crowning – it is beginning to emerge from the vaginal opening.

For most women the end of the transition stage is marked by a noticeable change in the pattern of breathing. You may grunt involuntarily, and this is because you will start to feel the urge to bear down. The need to push becomes very strong. Do tell your assistant to alert the staff that you are ready to push. They will confirm that the cervix has dilated 10 centimetres and the second stage is beginning. Your baby is about to be born.

BACKACHE LABOUR

If your baby is in the posterior position, its head may be pressing against your sacrum. This usually results in a long, erratic labour accompanied by backache. In this position the baby's head is not properly flexed and a wider part presents. However, the baby usually rotates before passing through the birth canal and the birth itself is normal. If your backache is particularly bad, there are ways to relieve it.

● Keep moving, and during contractions take up a position in which the pressure is

taken off your back, for example on all fours, leaning into a chair, or rocking to and fro.
● Nullify the pressure with counterpressure. Your birth assistant can apply pressure with fists or something round such as a tennis ball against your back.
● Apply a hot water bottle to the lower part of your back between contractions.
● Don't lie flat on your back; the baby's head then presses onto your spine.
● Massage the buttocks and the lower back (see p. 105).

POSITIONS DURING THE TRANSITION

Transition is a difficult stage in which to find a comfortable position. Contractions seem relentless but if you understand that the baby will be born soon, that should give you the encouragement and confidence to stay calm and patient. You probably won't feel like moving around so much but try to change positions every now and again.

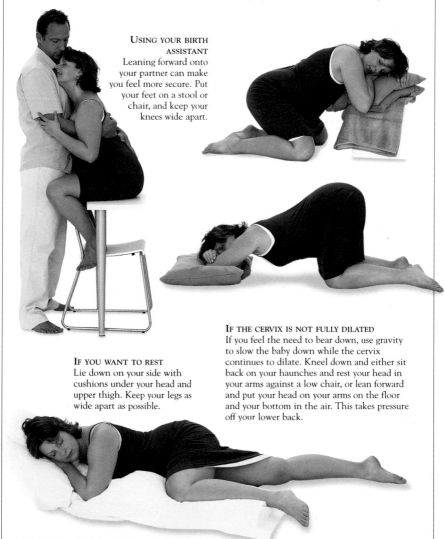

USING YOUR BIRTH ASSISTANT
Leaning forward onto your partner can make you feel more secure. Put your feet on a stool or chair, and keep your knees wide apart.

IF THE CERVIX IS NOT FULLY DILATED
If you feel the need to bear down, use gravity to slow the baby down while the cervix continues to dilate. Kneel down and either sit back on your haunches and rest your head in your arms against a low chair, or lean forward and put your head on your arms on the floor and your bottom in the air. This takes pressure off your lower back.

IF YOU WANT TO REST
Lie down on your side with cushions under your head and upper thigh. Keep your legs as wide apart as possible.

POSITIONS FOR DELIVERY

You will know by now from your experience of labour what position will be most comfortable to give birth in. Take advice from your medical attendants; they will lead you through the pushing stage. Enjoy yourself and take your time.

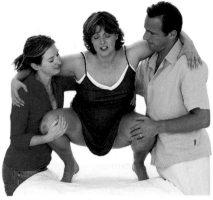

SUPPORTED SQUAT
Your partner can support you by taking your weight on his arms. He should keep his back straight, and his knees slightly bent.

SQUATTING
This opens up the pelvis, relaxes the pelvic floor and vaginal opening and uses the force of gravity to deliver the baby. To squat on a bed, you will need two helpers to support you so that you feel safe.

A COMMON DELIVERY POSITION
Sit propped up with cushions, hold onto your knees and drop your chin on your chest. You can lie back and relax between each contraction and conserve your energy. You will be able to see the baby emerge.

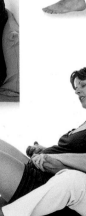

SEMI-UPRIGHT POSITION
If you feel happier being close to your partner during the delivery, you can lean back against him. His closeness will give you confidence and he can encourage you to push during contractions.

The second stage

FOR A FIRST BABY the second stage generally doesn't last longer than two hours – the average is around one hour and it may be as little as 5 minutes even for a first baby. Bearing down is a reflex action, an instinctive urge to push down, which is caused by the baby's head pressing on the pelvic floor and the rectum. Even if you know nothing about

ADVICE TO BIRTH ASSISTANT

● Remind her to relax her pelvic floor during pushing. She should take two or three deep breaths and push her hardest at the peak of contractions. She should push in a strong, steady way.
● Remind her to look in the mirror so that she can see the baby emerging.
● If you are in hospital and are asked to leave the delivery room suddenly, do so without question. There may be a medical emergency and staff will have to move very fast. You cannot guarantee that you will not be in the way. Leave the delivery room but stay close to outside.
● Remind her to lie back and relax fully between contractions so that she conserves her strength for pushing.
● You are now more of an observer once the baby's head has crowned. The midwife will be the one who coaches your partner through the pushing stage.
● Don't expect your partner to communicate with you during the birth. She will be preoccupied and may not notice you for some time.
● When the baby is placed on your partner's stomach, if possible put your arms around them both to keep them warm and signal that you're still there.
● Be ready for your own and your partner's reactions. There may be tears, silence, whoops of joy, perhaps even squeamishness. It's all perfectly normal and understandable so don't feel you have to hold back your emotions.

the mechanics of labour you will know automatically to take a deep breath, so lowering your diaphragm which exerts pressure on the uterus and helps the pushing. You then hold your breath, slightly bend your knees and strain downwards. Pushing is instinctive. It doesn't hurt the baby but it is quite hard work, and much harder work if you are lying on your back because you actually have to push the baby uphill (see p. 36). It is much less difficult if you are in an upright position, squatting, sitting up supported, on all fours, or on your knees leaning against a chair or your partner. This way you have the force of gravity to help you. Your pushing should be smooth and continuous. All of the muscular effort should be down and out. It should be fairly slow and gradual so that the vaginal tissues and muscles are given time to stretch and accommodate your baby's head without tearing or making an episiotomy necessary. Even so, you can still tear.

You should push during a contraction. Your pushing effort only *helps* the uterus to expel the baby. The involuntary muscles of the uterus can expel the baby on their own. So you help most by beginning your pushing effort with the peak intensity of each contraction.

During pushing, the pelvic floor and the anal area should be as relaxed as possible, so you need to make a conscious effort to relax this part of your body (see p. 85). You may urinate or lose a little stool but don't be embarrassed; they are both very common. When you've finished a push you will find two slow, deep breaths helpful, but don't relax too quickly at the end of each contraction as the baby will maintain its forward progress if you relax slowly.

Between contractions rest as much as you can. Conserve your energy for the next push.Breathe steadily and deeply. Don't talk if you don't want to.

BIRTH

The first sign that the baby is coming is bulging of the anus and perineum. With each contraction more and more of the baby's head appears at the vaginal opening, though it may slip back slightly between contractions. After crowning, the head will be delivered in the next contraction or two.

It is normal to feel a stinging or burning sensation as the baby stretches the outlet of the birth canal. As soon as you feel it, stop bearing down, pant and allow the uterus to push the baby out on its own. As you stop pushing, try to go limp. Make a conscious effort to relax the muscles of the perineal floor (see p. 85). The burning or stinging sensation lasts for a short time and is immediately followed by a numb feeling as the baby's head stretches the vaginal tissues so thin that the nerves are blocked, having a natural anaesthetic effect. If the medical staff feel you are going to tear badly, this is the moment they may do an episiotomy (see p. 138). As the baby's head is delivered, you will feel a sensation like toothpaste coming out of a tube. Once the head has emerged, the midwife will check that the cord is not round the baby's neck (see p. 132).

When the head is delivered, the baby's back is uppermost; its face is pointing towards your rectum. Almost immediately, however, it will start to rotate its shoulders so that it is facing your right or left thigh. The direction depends on its position in the uterus. The midwife will wipe its eyes, nose and mouth with clean gauze, and remove any fluid from the nose and upper air passages. Now there may be a breathing space when the uterine contractions stop for a few minutes. When they restart, it's hardly necessary for you to push because within the next one or two contractions, the baby's shoulders will be born, followed by its body. Sometimes head and body are born in the one contraction. Occasionally the baby's shoulders don't come out easily. The midwife will call for urgent help and an episiotomy may be needed.

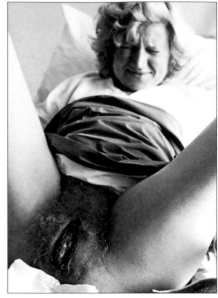

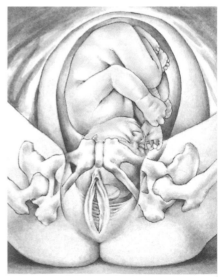

1 With each contraction in the second stage of labour, more of the baby's head appears at the vaginal opening. The anus and the perineum bulge out with the pressure of the head.

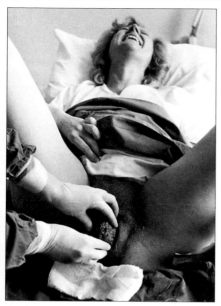

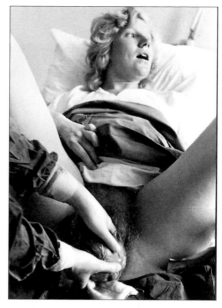

2 As the baby's head crowns, the stinging sensation is followed by numbness as the vaginal tissues are stretched so thin that the nerves are blocked. The head then slips out at last.

3 The baby's head is born facing downwards towards the rectum but the baby immediately turns to face your thigh to get into a good position for the birth of the body.

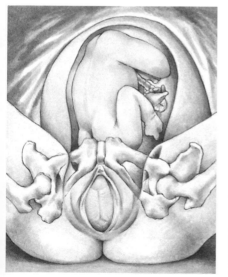

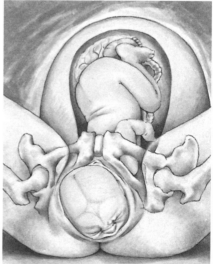

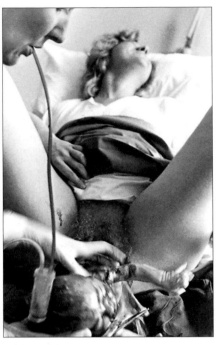

4 The midwife will clear mucus from the baby's air passages. The next contraction should be enough to deliver the shoulders. Then the baby is born and handed to the mother and the cord clamped and cut.

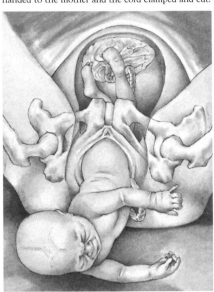

The midwife usually assists this last part of delivery by putting her thumbs and fingers under the armpits of your baby and lifting him upwards towards your abdomen, holding him firmly as he will be slippery with blood and amniotic fluid. If you're feeling alert and you're in a position to do so, you can bend down and pull your baby out yourself and onto your abdomen.

Your baby may cry when first delivered and will be crying lustily a few seconds after birth. If the breathing is normal, there's absolutely no reason why you should not take hold of the baby immediately. Ask if you can lay the baby on your abdomen and keep him warm with your arms and those of your partner. If there's a danger of the baby being cold, all three of you can be kept warm with a warm towel or blanket. Your gentle stroking movements, your soothing voice and the sound of your heartbeat are all right for your baby.

Your baby will probably be a bluish colour at first and may be covered with the white greasy vernix. He will have streaks of blood on his head and body and depending on your delivery his head may be elongated after the journey down the birth canal. The midwife will make a check of his general condition. If there is fluid in the mouth or nose or air passages, the midwife will want to make sure that it's cleared and breathing is normal. She will suck it out. If the baby doesn't start to breathe immediately, the midwife will take him and give him oxygen. Don't be alarmed at the sudden activity. As soon as the baby's breathing is normal, he will be returned to you to hold.

The third stage

WHEN THE BABY IS BORN the uterus rests and after about 15 minutes starts to contract comparatively painlessly again to expel the placenta. This is the third stage of labour. When the shoulder appears the midwife usually gives the mother an injection in the thigh of syntometrine or ergometrine, a synthetic hormone that increases the contractions of the uterus to prevent major haemorrhage. Oxytocin, produced naturally in response to seeing and touching your baby, but most of all to putting him to the breast, does the same job. The injection is usually administered in a hospital delivery, although the midwife or doctor will ask you first.

In the third stage of labour the placenta detaches itself from the uterine wall. The large blood vessels, about the thickness of a pencil, that run to and from the placenta are simply torn across. Most women do not bleed, however, because the muscle fibres of the uterus are arranged in a criss-cross fashion, and when the uterus contracts down, the muscles tighten around the blood vessels, preventing them from bleeding. This is why it's absolutely essential that the uterus contracts down into a hard ball once the placenta has been expelled. The uterus can be kept tightly contracted by massaging it for an hour or so after the third stage is complete.

The placenta slips out with a gentle squelch. It looks rather like a piece of liver and many women like to look at it and examine it. It is an amazing organ – it has been the life support system for your baby for nine months. Once the placenta is delivered, the midwife will examine it to make sure that none of it has been left behind. If any of the placenta has been retained by the uterus it can be a cause of haemorrhage later on and may need to be surgically removed.

You may shiver profoundly after delivery of the placenta. After delivery of my second child I was shivering so much and my teeth were chattering so that I couldn't speak and couldn't breathe properly. My explanation for this reaction is that for nine months I had a little furnace inside me, producing a lot of heat, and my body had adjusted to take account of that heat production by turning my own thermostat down slightly. When my baby left my body, I was deprived of that heat and I started shivering to raise my body temperature. The shivering usually passes in about half an hour, during which time the body temperature has been brought back up to normal and your own thermostat reset. Often the muscles in the legs feel quite sore for a day or two.

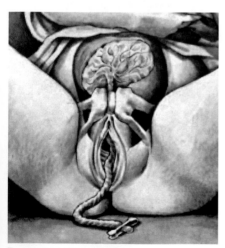

DELIVERY OF THE PLACENTA
When the contractions resume, they will be less painful. One or two pushes should expel the placenta. The midwife will put one hand on your uterus and will gently pull on the cord with the other to ease the placenta out.

CLAMPING THE CORD

There is no need for the unseemly rush to clamp the cord that there used to be 30 years ago when I first qualified. The cord will only need to be clamped and cut

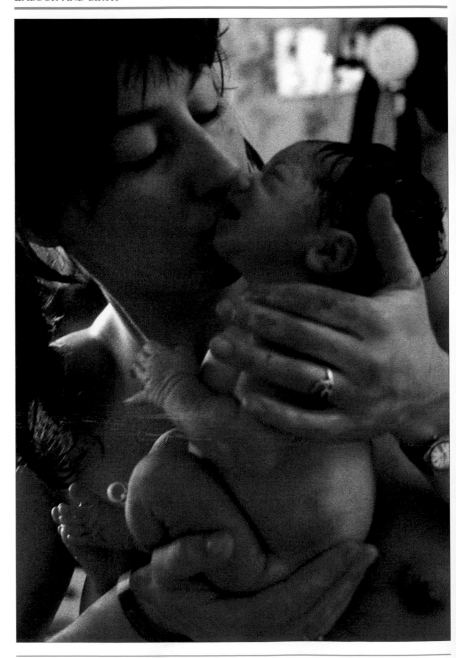

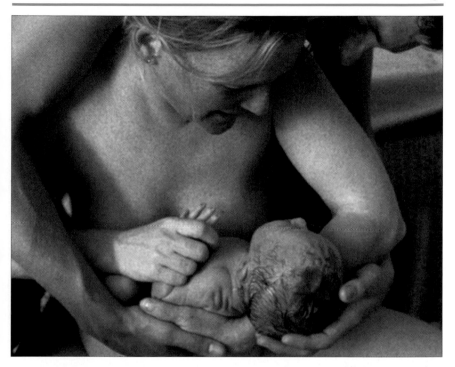

at once if it is looped tightly around the baby's neck. This is quite common, and the baby will then be delivered very quickly. Usually the midwife will be able to slip the cord out from around the baby's head and the delivery can proceed without immediate clamping. It's generally believed that the baby benefits from the return of placental blood through the umbilical cord and that it should not be clamped until it stops pulsating. (Blood can flow from the placenta to the baby only if the baby is at a lower level than the uterus.) When the time is right, the cord is divided between a pair of clamps placed 13–15cm (5–6in) from the baby's navel.

Now the three of you should be left alone. Put your baby to the breast as soon as possible – preferably in the first five minutes and even before the cord is clamped if that's an option. Breastfeeding releases oxytocin which helps the uterus

HOLDING YOUR BABY
While the placenta is being expelled, you can hold your baby for the first time.

to contract, and the colostrum in your breasts contains antibodies that will guard against some forms of gastric infection. Don't worry if he doesn't want to suckle, just concentrate on getting to know him. A newborn is usually alert during the first hour after a normal birth, and will look intently at you if you hold him 20–25cm (8–10in) from your face. He can focus at this distance, which is the distance between your face and his when you cradle him to the breast.

Presently you will be washed, stitched if necessary and asked to pass urine to check that everything is working all right. The midwives will wipe the baby and weigh him and put him in the crib ready for transferral to the postnatal ward.

Pain relief in labour

FEW LABOURS ARE PAINLESS but stories about suffering in labour are often exaggerated and distorted, and some women feel that severe pain is so inevitable that it becomes a self-fulfilling prophecy. The amount of pain actually felt almost always has a strong relationship to what is expected. Of course you should be realistic, but your expectations can be greatly modified by what you learn, the information you are given, and how confident you feel when you go into labour. This is why antenatal classes and breathing exercises, which give you the knowledge that you have some control over your body, and therefore some control over pain, are so important to you.

Everyone agrees that fear and ignorance cause tension, stress and anxiety, all of which make pain worse, and may even create pain where there is very little. Information, knowledge and support can go a long way to dispel fear and anxiety, and will also help to ease pain. There's no question that pain can be relieved with drugs, but to my mind the best form of pain relief is information, a calm state of mind and moral support. Armed with these you will find not only that the pain you feel is less, but that you may be strong enough to cope with it without resorting to analgesics or anaesthetics which might dim your consciousness and awareness of what's going on – something that most women these days want to avoid.

Doctors and midwives believe that an important part of their job is to make labour as pain-free as possible and if they feel you are in difficulty they will be keen to offer you a range of analgesics. However, they will not force anything on you. It is a good idea to discuss pain relief at the antenatal clinic early in your pregnancy, to make your preferences clear (see p. 46) and have them recorded in your notes and birth plan. Remember to state alternatives in case things don't go according to plan.

Of course it's impossible to know your own pain threshold in advance and not all problems can be predicted. So it is important to go into labour with an open mind and to accept the pain relief offered if it is considered essential. Whatever happens, don't feel guilty; not everyone has a trouble-free labour and birth.

DECISION TO ACCEPT PAIN RELIEF

There are two important considerations about the use of painkilling drugs in labour. With most drugs, whether they're sedatives which make you feel calm and sleepy, hypnotics which actually send you to sleep, or narcotics which make you feel light-headed and cut off from the normal world, you will lose some awareness of what is happening around you. Many women want to experience every second of giving birth and any interference with their level of awareness is unacceptable. The second important factor is that most drugs will cross the placenta to the baby and will be in a higher concentration in the baby's blood than in the mother's blood. Many mothers find this unacceptable. Bearing both of these things in mind, and after getting as much information as you need, make up your mind about your attitude to having painkilling drugs in your labour.

A useful tip is to wait a little before accepting drugs. Some good news and moral support may be enough to get you over a sticky patch. Ask how far dilated you are. If you feel you are making good progress and can hang on, that may increase your resolve. Some encouraging words from your partner will give you added strength. So give yourself about 15 minutes after you feel you may want some pain relief before actually having it. During that time you may make quite good progress. You may even have got through the most painful parts of labour and have only a little way to go. You may be astonished at your own strength and resilience and feel that you can manage perfectly well without drugs.

ANALGESICS

Analgesics are drugs that relieve pain. They work by numbing the pain centre of the brain. Inhalation analgesia (sometimes erroneously known as gas and air) is in fact a mixture of nitrous oxide and oxygen called Entonox. It is self-administered and you can inhale it half a minute before the peak of a contraction. You may become light-headed while inhaling it, but regain full consciousness a few seconds later. You will be given the opportunity to practise with the machine in your antenatal classes. Even if you don't use it successfully during labour, it gives you something to concentrate on while you are having contractions; this can be quite useful if you're becoming discouraged.

Pethidine is a narcotic given by injection in varying dosages during the first stage. It takes about 20 minutes to work and is sometimes combined with other drugs. Pethidine relaxes you and relieves your anxiety but its painkilling effect is variable. It is given less frequently than it used to be largely because it was used to relieve maternal fatigue if the first stage of labour was protracted. With modern aids, mothers no longer become overtired and distressed in the way they used to. The safest time to administer the drug is six to eight hours before delivery. As this is difficult to calculate and the drug wears off in about two hours, it is probably best for those women who are nervous and anxious during the early first stage of labour.

ENTONOX
Used properly, Entonox, also known as gas and air, gives a mild level of pain relief. It can be delivered via a demand valve, as here, or through a face mask.

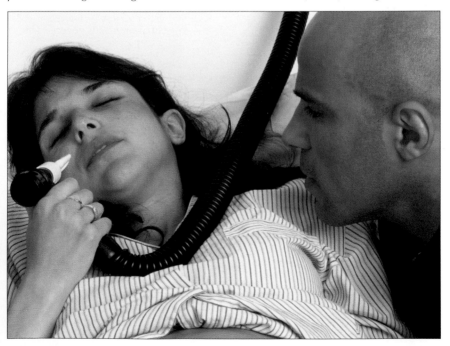

ANAESTHETICS

A general anaesthetic is never used during a normal birth, but a local or regional anaesthetic may be given to dull your conscious appreciation of pain. Anaesthetic is injected into a nerve root to numb the part of the body which the nerve supplies. The most widely used local anaesthetic is the epidural (see right). There is also the pudendal block, a local anaesthetic injection to numb the lower part of the vagina before forceps or ventouse deliveries. A needle is guided through the vagina to make an injection round the pudendal nerve.

EPIDURAL ANAESTHESIA

The epidural, which has been called the Cadillac of anaesthetics, prevents pain being felt in the abdominal area by acting as a "nerve block" in the spine. It probably has no effect on the fetus directly but it does affect you in labour. One of the reasons why the epidural has become so popular is that it fulfils all the criteria of a good pain reliever but in no way interferes with your awareness and your levels of consciousness. There are very few side effects associated with the majority of epidural anaesthetics, and for many women it is a perfect answer.

HAVING AN EPIDURAL

An epidural takes about 10–20 minutes for a skilled anaesthetist to set up. The analgesic effect is usually felt in just a few minutes and lasts for about two hours but you can be "topped up" when the pain returns and becomes severe.

SETTING UP AN EPIDURAL
You will be asked to empty your bladder before lying down on your left side and pulling your legs up to make as tight a ball as possible. Your lower back will be washed with cold spirit and then you will be given an injection of local anaesthetic. A small hole will be made in your back with a solid needle and a hollow needle is then inserted in its place. Once the epidural space is located, a fine catheter is threaded through the hollow needle and into the epidural space, leaving a length of catheter protruding from your back. The catheter is secured to your skin along its length with paper tape. The local anaesthetic is then given by syringe down the catheter and the opening is sealed. You will have a drip set up so that fluids can be fed to you intravenously should your blood pressure fall.

THE POSITION FOR SETTING UP THE EPIDURAL

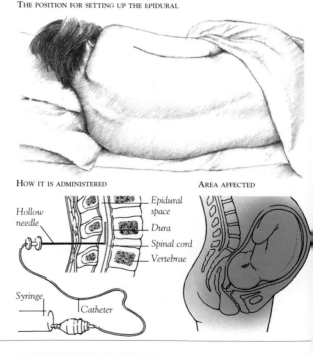

HOW IT IS ADMINISTERED

Hollow needle

Syringe

Catheter

Epidural space
Dura
Spinal cord
Vertebrae

AREA AFFECTED

HYPNOSIS

Hypnosis can relieve pain in a susceptible person. However, many practice sessions during pregnancy are advisable and both you and the hypnotist (see p. 154) should be familiar with what is required of you.

ACUPUNCTURE

I would recommend using acupuncture for pain relief in labour only if you have found it successful in the past. For some women it will undoubtedly work but the acupuncturist (see p. 155) must be practised at giving pain relief in labour.

TENS

TENS stands for transcutaneous nerve stimulation and is a means of relieving labour pain by stimulating production of the body's natural painkillers – endorphins – and by blocking pain sensation with an electric current. The electrodes are placed on the woman's body and she is able to regulate the intensity of the current herself. TENS has been used successfully but it does not help everyone, particularly not those women who experience lots of pain. TENS doesn't relieve all of the pain but what remains is possibly easier to bear. A try-out before labour is advisable.

ADVANTAGES AND DISADVANTAGES OF AN EPIDURAL

ADVANTAGES

1 An epidural provides complete pain relief without dulling any of your mental faculties.
2 It has a tendency to slow down labour which can be useful.
3 No other local anaesthetic will be necessary should you need forceps, vacuum extraction or episiotomy at the last minute.
4 It allows you to participate in your birth if you have a Caesarean, and the baby needs less resuscitation than with a general anaesthetic.
5 As it lowers blood pressure it is ideal for women with pre-eclampsia or high blood pressure.
6 It can be topped up with extra anaesthetic or allowed to wear off near the delivery so that you can control the actual birth. The contractions at this stage may be a bit of a shock, though, if you haven't experienced any until then.
7 It reduces the amount of work done by the lungs in labour and so can benefit women who suffer from any form of heart or lung disease.

DISADVANTAGES

1 The lowering of blood pressure may make you feel dizzy and nauseous. This is more likely if you lie on your back so turn onto your side.
2 There is the possibility of a post-anaesthetic headache which lasts a few hours after delivery.
3 There is a possibility of an episiotomy and a forceps delivery. Depending on the concentration of the anaesthetic, there may be a loss of muscle power and of the sensation of the contractions. This results in a slower second stage because you will be entirely dependent on the instructions of the midwife as to when to push the baby out. The length of the second stage is the factor that determines whether or not forceps are used
4 If the mother's blood pressure drops, the amount of blood supplying the placenta is reduced and so the oxygen supply to the baby is lowered.
5 If an epidural is allowed to wear off near delivery, the contractions may come as a nasty shock.
6 Not all epidurals are effective.

PAIN RELIEF IN LABOUR

TYPE OF DRUG	ACTION	EFFECT ON MOTHER & BABY
NARCOTICS (morphine, pethidine)	Sedate and relieve anxiety. Possibly relieve pain during the first stage of labour.	Reduce consciousness and tend to make the labour longer. Cross the placenta in five minutes and can depress respiration at birth. Sucking may be inefficient (see p. 145). Can produce nausea in the mother.
INHALATION ANALGESIA (Entonox)	Relieves pain. Can cause drowsiness if allowed to accumulate.	Depresses alertness but this returns once the effects have worn off. Makes you lightheaded while breathing in the gas. No significant effect on the baby.

Medical intervention

DURING THE LAST 20 years hospital childbirth has been revolutionized by the development of new procedures which have been widely adopted as routine practice. All offer advantages; a few carry risks, though small. None of them should be used unless there are good medical reasons. Most people believe that the convenience of the staff or even of the mother should not be the sole justification for the employment of these procedures.

EPISIOTOMY

In an episiotomy, which takes place during the second stage of labour, an incision is made in the perineum between the vaginal opening and the anus to facilitate delivery of the baby. It is the most common operation in the western world.

The cut is made with scissors under a local anaesthetic just as the baby's head appears. If it is done too early, before the perineum has thinned out, muscles, skin and blood vessels are damaged and the bleeding may be profuse. Also the tissues are crushed by the scissors as they are cut. This leads to bruising, swelling and slow healing and accounts for a great deal of

the pain and discomfort which often follows episiotomy. There is also the possibility that the integrity of the pelvic floor can be damaged if the muscle fibres are not correctly aligned. If the vagina and perineum are stitched too tightly a woman may experience discomfort when intercourse is resumed. You might like to

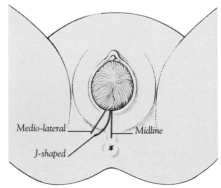

EPISIOTOMY INCISIONS
The different types of incision include the medio-lateral, from the back of the vagina out to the side; the midline, which runs between the vagina and the anus; and the J-shaped cut, which combines the two.

have it recorded in your notes that you wish to avoid having an episiotomy if it is at all possible.

If medical staff indicate that they think an episiotomy is necessary during labour, you should ask why it's being done.

AVOIDING AN EPISIOTOMY

One of the best ways to avoid the necessity for an episiotomy is to deliver your baby in as upright a position as you possibly can (see p. 36). Tell your midwife early in labour that you want to find a good position for the second stage of labour and in particular that you'd like to avoid lying on your back. Together with your birth partner, your midwife will then be ready to help give you the support you need when the time comes.

If you learn how to relax the muscles of the pelvic floor antenatally and allow your vaginal tissues and perineum to bulge out (see p. 85) you can probably avoid a tear. Familiarity with the sensation when the baby's head bulges or "crowns" will mean that you will realize that you are starting to tighten up in the second stage and you can try to do something about it. Having an epidural anaesthetic may increase the possibility of having an

episiotomy. If you do opt for an epidural, there is no reason why an episiotomy is automatically necessary, but you will need to make your views known to your midwife and birth partner.

It is also a good idea to try to have the end of the second stage well under your control by relaxing the pelvic floor muscle and not pushing down too hard when the baby's head is delivered. I had an epidural twice, but on neither occasion did I have an episiotomy.

EXPERIENCE OF EPISIOTOMY

Sheila Kitzinger, in her study of 2000 women who had episiotomies, came to the following conclusions:
• Episiotomies were more painful than a tear.
• Women found it more difficult to get into a comfortable position to hold the baby after an episiotomy.
• The pain distracted them during breastfeeding.
• An episiotomy was more likely to give pain or discomfort during sexual intercourse even three months after delivery.
• Two-thirds of the women had never discussed episiotomy with medical staff during pregnancy. Some had tried but had been unsuccessful.
• About half the episiotomies had been done when the perineum was not sufficiently thinned out.
• More than half the women had not been instructed to release the vagina and pelvic floor muscles but had been encouraged to push instead, which made the episiotomy more necessary.
• About one-quarter of the women had not been told to stop pushing while the head was being born to give the vagina a chance to thin out.
• More than a third of the women were never given a reason for the episiotomy.
• Some women found the stitching painful but when they complained they were told (incorrectly) that there were no nerve endings there.

REASONS FOR AN EPISIOTOMY

An episiotomy will be necessary if:
• The perineum hasn't had time to stretch slowly – breathing exercises and massage help with this.
• The baby's head is too large for the vaginal opening.
• You aren't able to control your pushing so that you can stop when necessary and then push gradually and smoothly. An episiotomy will deliver the baby quickly if you have difficulty with co-ordination and control of pushing in the second stage.
• The baby is distressed.
• You have a forceps or ventouse (vacuum extraction) delivery.
• Yours is a breech birth.

INDUCTION

Induction is the artificial "starting off" of labour. Your labour will be induced should it fail to start on its own or if for some reason your doctor decides that you need to deliver the baby early.

Induction is usually planned in advance; depending on the hospital, you may be admitted the night before or you may simply come into the hospital on the day. Induction is often introduced gradually, first with prostaglandin pessaries, then if necessary, by rupturing the membranes (ARM), and finally, if things are going too slowly, with an oxytocin drip.

PROSTAGLANDIN PESSARIES

No one knows exactly why labour starts but pessaries or a gel containing prostaglandins, which are made up of various hormones that have an effect on a pregnant woman's uterus, are used to induce labour.

The use of prostaglandin pessaries is the least invasive method of starting labour. Pessaries are inserted into the vagina, and labour will usually start within a few hours. Sometimes a single pesssary may be enough, but more than one may be needed to get things going. In 50 per cent of cases the prostaglandin pessaries may be supplemented with ARM and an oxytocin drip.

ARTIFICIAL RUPTURE OF THE MEMBRANES

Also known as ARM or amniotomy, rupturing the membranes is only done if the cervix is sufficiently open and the head is low in the pelvis. It doesn't in itself stimulate contractions although they may start spontaneously. However, ARM often needs supplementing with oxytocin to stimulate contractions, because labour must begin within 24 hours to avoid the risk of infection.

A pair of forceps or a tool not unlike a crochet hook is inserted into the womb and a small opening is made in the membrane so that the waters escape. For most women this is a painless procedure. Labour usually reaches full intensity quickly after ARM because the baby's head is no longer cushioned and presses hard against the cervix, encouraging the uterus to contract.

Amniotomy was until fairly recently almost a routine procedure during the preparation for any labour. If left alone, the waters may rupture spontaneously at any stage of labour. There are two major disadvantages of amniotomy. The first is that it makes the labour proceed more intensely than it would normally. Also, if the baby has the cord around its neck, the loss of fluid increases pressure and can affect the flow of blood through the cord to the baby.

AMNIOTOMY
The bag of waters usually ruptures naturally towards the end of the first stage of labour. Before it breaks, it provides a cushion for the baby's head as it presses against the cervix (right). Once the membranes have ruptured (far right), the contractions increase in intensity because the baby's head is now resting hard against the cervix. This speeds up labour, which is why amniotomy may be performed if progress is slow.

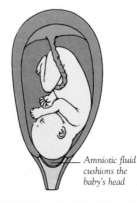

Amniotic fluid cushions the baby's head

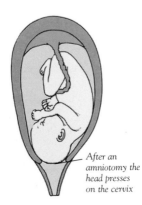

After an amniotomy the head presses on the cervix

Besides being a method of induction, amniotomy will be performed if an electrode is to be attached to the baby's head to monitor its heartbeat (see p. 142); if the baby's heart rate goes down, the amniotic fluid can be examined for traces of meconium, the first bowel movements of the baby. Meconium in the fluid can indicate fetal distress.

OXYTOCIN-INDUCED LABOUR

The hormone oxytocin, which is produced by the pituitary gland in the brain, stimulates the uterus to start contracting. It is therefore given in a synthetic form to start labour off and to keep it going.

Oxytocin is normally given via a drip inserted into a vein. Ask for it to be inserted in the arm you use least and check that you have a long tube connecting you to the drip. You should then have more room to move around, even if just on the bed. The drip can be turned down if you go into strong labour quickly and the cervix becomes half dilated. The needle won't be removed from your arm until after the baby is born as the uterus needs to keep contracting to expel the placenta and then prevent bleeding (see p. 131).

The contractions you experience while on an oxytocin drip are often stronger, longer and more painful, with shorter periods of relaxation in between. Unfortunately this may mean the need for painkilling drugs is greater. Also, the blood supply to the uterus is temporarily shut off during each strong contraction, which may be detrimental to the baby.

REASONS FOR INDUCTION

Forty years ago induction was frequently used for hospital or social convenience. Induction was sometimes planned to suit working hours or changes in shifts, for example. In the sixties and seventies, obstetrics went through a phase of over-zealous high-tech intervention, when there was a great vogue for induced labours, especially in older mothers who, at that time, were much less common than today. Oxytocin-induced labour was once used in as many as 40–50 per cent of deliveries. Given that the rate of success with this form of induction is only about 85 per cent, its routine use cannot be justified, and most modern obstetricians believe that less than a few per cent of pregnant women require it. Nowadays fewer than one in five labours are induced by any method and I'd like to reassure you that induction is a great asset provided it's done strictly for medical reasons, such as pre-eclampsia.

Only five per cent of babies actually come on the due date and it's hard for some doctors and quite a lot of mothers to remain philosophical when that magic date passes. Both are concerned in case the baby is "postmature", or late. The fear is that the placenta may be becoming inadequate to support the baby and the baby is outgrowing its food supply.

Very few babies are truly overdue, however; 80 per cent of all babies who are born with a spontaneous labour arrive after the due date. This is mainly because medical convention calculates the expected date of delivery from the last menstrual period rather than from the time of conception (see p. 21). Most doctors accept that up to 14 days after the expected date is normal.

Many units now offer induction at ten days after term and recommend it at 14 days after term because of the risk of late stillbirth. After 14 days, signs of postmaturity are carefully looked for. Screening involves monitoring the fetal heart and movements and ultrasound for amniotic fluid measurement.

However, waiting until the expected day of delivery is leaving it a bit late to face the prospect of an induced labour. This is something that should be read about and discussed earlier in pregnancy and you and your doctor should try to agree on the course to be followed should induction be necessary in your case.

ELECTRONIC FETAL MONITORING

Electronic fetal monitoring (EFM) is a method of recording the baby's heartbeat and your contractions during labour. It is the high-tech replacement for the ear trumpet or fetoscope, but has by no means superseded these. Almost all maternity units ask you to be monitored routinely for about 20 minutes, but if all is well there is no need for you to be continuously monitored.

Monitoring is usually done with belts strapped around your abdomen that simultaneously pick up contractions and the baby's heartbeat, recording them on a graph. The print-out can then be interpreted by the midwife to make sure that the baby's heart is beating normally during the contraction (see below right). During a contraction blood flow to your placenta is reduced for a few seconds and your baby's heart rate dips. It then returns to normal when the contraction passes. Occasionally doctors may think it necessary to attach an electrode to the baby's scalp as well, if the abdominal recording is of poor quality and your baby is thought to need constant

FETAL MONITOR ELECTRODE

If your medical team think that your baby needs closer monitoring, they may want to attach an electrode to his head. Once your cervix is at least 2–3 centimetres dilated, you will be given an amniotomy to break your waters (see p. 140) if they haven't broken already. An electrode is then attached to the part of the baby that is going to be born first, which is usually his head. The electrode pierces the skin slightly and provides an electrical contact that tracks the baby's heartbeat. Electronic signals are then relayed to the external monitor and a graph is printed out for the staff to interpret.

monitoring. The electrode is attached to his presenting part, usually to the skin on the top of his head, and picks up his heartbeat. It is an accurate method of monitoring, but it does mean that your waters will have to be broken if they haven't already done so.

MONITORING IN LABOUR
Many women find the monitor reassuring. They can see the contractions coming and prepare for them and they can watch their baby's heartbeat throughout labour.

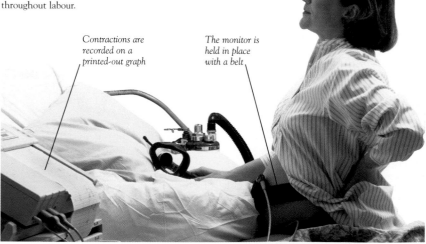

Contractions are recorded on a printed-out graph

The monitor is held in place with a belt

CONTINUOUS EFM

Monitoring the baby's heartbeat and the uterine contractions is essential if you are being induced (see p. 140), if your labour is being accelerated or if you have an epidural, when you will be less able to feel the onset of contractions. Most hospitals now agree that EFM should be used routinely in high-risk pregnancies.

Electronic fetal monitoring involving a fetal scalp electrode used to confine mothers to bed but nowadays it is less restricting. A method of monitoring by radio waves, known as telemetry, allows the mother to walk about away from the monitoring equipment. The electrode is still attached to the baby's head but it is joined to a strap on the mother's thigh and not to a large machine. However, babies do suffer rashes where the electrode was clipped to them and there is no proof that they feel no pain. Electronic fetal monitoring provides the medical staff with a second-by-second report

PROBLEMS WITH CONTINUOUS EFM

● The staff are more aware of any small changes and may therefore be more likely to intervene rather than letting labour take its natural course.
● Babies who are electronically monitored are three times more likely to be delivered by Caesarean section.
● EFM increases the electronic paraphernalia in the delivery room.
● Staff may be tempted to concentrate more on the machine than on the woman in labour.
● EFM may restrict movement, thus slowing down the labour and making fetal distress more likely.
● Attaching the electrode may bruise and hurt the baby's head.

on the condition of your baby, so that they can intervene quickly if he is in distress. If a doctor tells you that you need continuous EFM, try to see that as reassuring, because it will ensure that you get the best possible care for your baby.

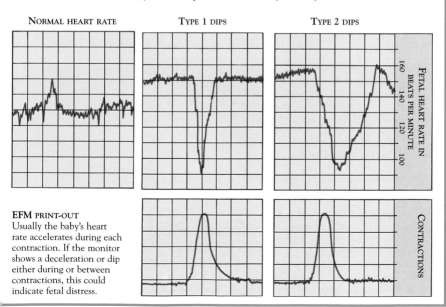

NORMAL HEART RATE   TYPE 1 DIPS   TYPE 2 DIPS

FETAL HEART RATE IN BEATS PER MINUTE

160 140 120 100

CONTRACTIONS

EFM PRINT-OUT
Usually the baby's heart rate accelerates during each contraction. If the monitor shows a deceleration or dip either during or between contractions, this could indicate fetal distress.

12

Complications surrounding the birth

Even the best planned labours may not go according to plan,
especially for first-time mothers. You may become exhausted or your
baby may become distressed and need to be delivered quickly. Thinking
about the possibility of a Caesarean or forceps delivery in advance will
help you to know what to expect should the situation arise.

Breech birth

A BREECH BABY is one that is born
buttocks first. Most babies move around
freely until about the 32nd week of
pregnancy when they turn head down
(cephalic position). Four out of every
hundred babies, however, stay put. If your
baby is one of these, do not be concerned;
most breech labours are smooth, though
you will have to have the baby in
hospital. Doctors used to try to turn
breech babies by applying gentle external
pressure on the abdomen. This procedure
is rarely performed now.

Doctors do not generally recommend a
home birth if the baby is in the breech
position. However, if you are at home, try
to adopt a supported upright position with
your legs wide apart and your knees bent
to give the baby's head more space.

After the birth, your genital region
might be slightly swollen but the swelling
will subside within 48 hours. Because
many breech births are helped by forceps,
babies may have bruises on the face and
head, but they will fade fast. You are more
likely to have an episiotomy (see p. 138)

with a breech birth because the head has
less time to be compressed during delivery,
making it more likely to get stuck.

Attitudes towards breech births differ:
some doctors feel that a breech baby
should always be delivered by Caesarean
section, others are less rigid. However,
about 80 per cent of breech babies are
delivered by Caesarean section in the UK.

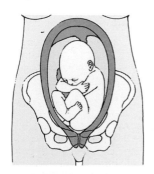

A WELL-FLEXED BREECH BABY
It is possible to deliver a baby in this position
vaginally, though an episiotomy may be necessary.

BIRTH OF A BREECH BABY

The baby's buttocks press against the cervix and effacement and dilatation of the cervix occur as with a cephalic presentation (see p. 120). The waters usually break early with a breech presentation and you will probably feel contractions as bad backache (see p. 124). Kneeling on all fours is a helpful position to relieve this during the first stage. For the birth, the supported squatting position is safest and an episiotomy may be done in this position if necessary, though your doctor may prefer the lithotomy position (see p. 36). Sometimes forceps may be used to protect the baby's head during delivery. Epidurals are advised to prevent pushing before the cervix is fully dilated. If you then need a Caesarean section, this will save time and allow you to hold your baby the moment he is born.

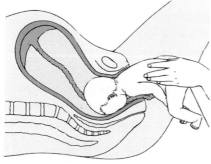

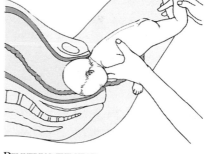

DELIVERING THE BODY
The buttocks are delivered first and then the legs. While the body is being delivered, it is better to breathe through the contractions than to push. Before the head is delivered you may be given an episiotomy, and forceps are inserted at this point.

DELIVERING THE HEAD
The weight of the baby's body draws the head down to the vagina and the body is then lifted to deliver the head. Doctors usually use forceps to protect the head from too much compression, and one push is usually enough to deliver the baby.

Caesarean section

INEVITABLY THERE ARE slight risks, such as infection, bleeding and clot formation, associated with Caesarean section, as it is a major operation. There is also the disadvantage of being left with a scar on the uterus that may weaken it. The rate of Caesarean sections is still rising so there is some concern that the operation is undertaken without enough thought.

Caesarean sections are now usually done under an epidural, or spinal, anaesthetic (see p. 136), which is safer than a general anaesthetic for you and the baby and means you can be conscious throughout.

However, if an epidural isn't already in place at the time, an emergency Caesarean may have to be done under general anaesthetic.

You may know weeks or only days in advance that you are to have your baby by Caesarean section. This is known as a planned or "elective" Caesarean. You will be admitted to hospital on a certain day, but if you go into labour spontaneously beforehand, you will still be given a Caesarean. Some Caesareans are performed as emergencies when it's essential that the baby is delivered quickly.

PREPARING FOR A CAESAREAN

Some women find a Caesarean section a great disappointment after looking forward to a vaginal delivery, especially if the hospital unit is not one that allows mothers and fathers to participate actively in the Caesarean labour and birth, and have immediate and intimate contact with the baby at birth and afterwards. Some women feel guilty that they've let their partner down and that he couldn't be there with them at the time of birth. Many mothers are angered and disappointed if they're not able to have their baby with them after the operation and have to be separated just at the time when mother and baby need each other for mutual support. But these psychological effects can be minimized if you prepare yourself for having a Caesarean section and look on it as a positive experience.

Ask to see your obstetrician so that you and your partner can have a relaxed discussion about what the operation entails, what the procedures will be in the operating theatre, whether you can have epidural anaesthesia and be awake and alert during the operation and whether your partner can be with you.

Ask your hospital clinic if there is a video available that shows what happens during a Caesarean. You can also prepare yourself by talking to other women who have had Caesarean sections. This is one of the best ways of preventing you from having negative feelings about it. Not only will you get moral support but you'll also get useful information about what it feels like, how long it takes to be completely fit again after the operation and tips on caring for your baby while your wound is healing. By talking to mothers who've had subsequent pregnancies after a Caesarean section, you can allay your fears about the future. A self-help group will be able to put you in touch with midwives and obstetricians who have a flexible and realistic attitude to pregnancy after Caesarean section.

WHAT HAPPENS

Your pubic hair will be shaved, the epidural anaesthesia will be set up, you'll have an intravenous drip inserted into your arm so that fluids can be fed directly into your bloodstream, and a catheter will be inserted into your bladder to drain away urine. A screen will probably be placed in front of your face and your partner might prefer to stand behind it at your head if he doesn't want to see the surgical procedure. A Caesarean section usually takes about 45 minutes but the baby is delivered within the first 5–10 minutes. The remaining time is for stitching the uterine wall and the abdomen. A small horizontal incision is made (see below) and the amniotic fluid is then drained off by suction – you'll hear this quite clearly. The baby is then gently lifted out either by hand or with forceps. You will be given an injection of ergometrine to make the uterus contract and to prevent bleeding. You and your partner can hold the baby while the third stage is completed. If everything is all right you can start nursing him as soon as possible. Depending on the reasons for the operation, your baby may be taken away to special care for an observation period. The catheter and the drip will remain in for some hours and the stitches or clamps will be removed five days later.

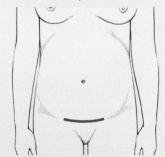

THE HORIZONTAL LINE INCISION
The so-called "bikini line" incision is common for obvious cosmetic reasons and because the low transverse cut heals more effectively.

REASONS FOR A CAESAREAN SECTION

- Fetus shows signs of profound distress; this will be obvious if the heart rate slows or "dips" at each contraction and, more seriously, between each contraction – this will show up on the print-out from the electronic monitors (see p. 142). If there is meconium in the amniotic fluid, the baby may have had a bowel movement which could indicate distress.
- The baby is extremely large or there may be cephalo-pelvic disproportion, where the baby's head is larger than the pelvic cavity.
- Breech babies (see p. 144) are often delivered by Caesarean section, particularly in the United States.
- A previous baby was born by this method; this is the commonest reason for the operation in the United States.
- Prolapse of the umbilical cord through the cervix.

- Placenta praevia.
- Abruptio placentae.
- The baby needs to be delivered early and induction and normal labour are considered to be an unnecessary risk to the baby or the mother.
- A serious infection of the vagina, such as a first-time attack of genital herpes.
- The cervix fails to dilate.
- Forceps fail to deliver the baby.
- Serious Rhesus incompatibility.

Some of the conditions that warrant abdominal delivery of the baby may not be apparent until labour has begun and this will then result in an emergency Caesarean section. Even so, many emergency sections are now performed under epidurals and do not require general anaesthetic. An alternative is a spinal anaesthetic (which is like an epidural but cannot be topped up).

Forceps delivery

ONE OF THE ARGUMENTS that has been put forward by the advocates of natural childbirth is that forceps are being commonly required because mothers are routinely given drugs and anaesthetics that interfere with their own efforts to deliver the baby. In other words, a certain proportion of forceps deliveries are probably doctor induced.

For centuries obstetric forceps offered the only method of delivering a baby that was not a natural delivery. As Caesarean section has become safer, the use of forceps has declined to the extent that they are no longer used for any hazardous type of delivery.

Nowadays, forceps are applied only when the first stage is complete, the cervix is fully dilated and the baby's head has descended well into the mother's pelvis but has failed to descend any further, or there are signs of either fetal or maternal distress.

A forceps delivery normally takes place with the mother in the lithotomy position (see p. 36). It can be done under an epidural or a local anaesthetic will be injected into the perineum. The forceps, which are shaped rather like serving tongs, are inserted into your vagina one side at a time. The doctor will have already determined where the baby's head lies and with gentle pulling on the forceps for 30–40 seconds at a time, and in time with your contractions, the baby's head gradually descends to the perineum. There should be little pain. An episiotomy (see p. 138) is then performed. When the head is delivered, the forceps are removed and the delivery can be completed normally.

If longer forceps are needed to pull the baby out, you may be given a pudendal nerve block, which is a local anaesthetic that is injected into the vaginal wall (see p. 136).

12

The first days

The birth of your baby is a climax to the nine months of waiting and anything that follows must, to a certain extent, fall in its shadow. During the first three days while you're waiting for the milk to come in, you may feel excited or tentative or you may find yourself in a state of shock. It's thrilling to explore your new baby and to enjoy quiet moments together, but don't be surprised if at times it feels like a bit of a let-down.

If you are in hospital for a few days after the birth, it's important to look and learn from the midwives and the experienced mothers on the ward. However, if you're a first-time mother, don't compare yourself with them and don't resent their experienced handling of their babies. The most important advice I can give you is to be easy on yourself. Don't try to be the perfect mother, and don't try to accomplish too much in these first days. You should remember to take one day at a time.

Bonding

IT'S DIFFICULT TO DESCRIBE what bonding is; it's certainly getting to know your baby and exploring her with your eyes, nose, ears, fingertips and mouth, and even your tongue. It's also to do with attachment, protectiveness and possessiveness. This early attachment is possibly the strongest bond between human beings, and necessarily so, as it ensures the nurturing of infants, and hence the survival of the human race.

Establishing a relationship with your baby begins the second she is born. If possible you should be left in private with your partner with a minimum of interruption for some time during the first hour after the birth. Research has shown that babies are usually quiet but very alert in the first hour of life, and in this state they are extremely responsive. They will stare intently at your face if held 20–25cm (8–10in) away. They can focus their eyes at this distance and respond to the human face. In addition, like most newborn animals, human babies have an instinct to bond with their parents. This is the right time for attachment to a caring adult, so both of you should make the most of it. Keep the lighting low and lay your baby against your body so that you make skin-to-skin contact. Looking into your baby's eyes renders her a person and not a thing, and skin contact allows you to feel each other as warm human beings.

The midwife may want to stitch you at this time, because early stitching is quicker and easier than if left until later, when the tissues may be swollen. It will probably be possible to hold your baby while it is being done or else your partner can have valuable one-to-one contact with his new baby. Other cleaning up can wait a while.

All aspects of the bonding process – your voice, smell, touch, caresses, fondling – are good for the baby, and they're also good for you. The sooner you touch and fondle your baby, the more quickly your bleeding will cease, the more strongly your uterus will contract and the better your breasts will respond with the let-down of colostrum and later milk. You are also increasing your confidence in handling the baby and helping her adapt to a new environment. Studies show that babies adapt more easily when they are held, soothed, crooned at and allowed to feed at will. Soon after you take hold of your baby, try putting her to your breast. Touch her cheek with your nipple and she will turn towards the breast. If she shows little perseverance – she may be sleepy if you had drugs for pain relief – express a little colostrum onto her lips to encourage her. Your partner can help by supporting the baby's head until you feel comfortable.

You may not bond instantly, however, particularly if you had a long or difficult labour. Don't worry; you have plenty of time to get to know your baby later.

THE FIRST HOUR OF LIFE
The sooner you start to touch and cuddle your baby the better for the bonding process, and you will help her adapt to her new world.

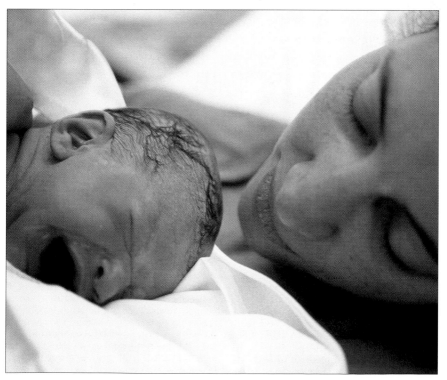

IMPORTANCE OF BONDING

If it seems that I'm emphasizing this bonding process between parent and infant, I feel it's for good reason. Research has shown that parents who are given unrestricted contact with their children immediately after delivery rear their children in a more constructive way, are more sympathetic to problems, ask more questions, give reasons for their actions, and explain situations better than do parents whose babies are taken away at birth. A further part of this research showed that at the age of five years the children who had had extended contact with their parents scored higher in intelligence tests than the control group. This does not mean that good bonding with your infant makes your baby a more intelligent child. What I think it points to is that it makes you a different kind of parent and possibly a better one.

FATHER'S FIRST CONTACT

Paternal bonding with an infant is not very different and certainly just as important as maternal bonding. So during this sensitive period after the birth it's important for you to hold your baby and make eye and skin contact. If you have been present at the birth and comforted your partner throughout the labour, this is a good beginning. Stay with your partner and your baby as long as possible after the birth. Be responsive to the cues that your infant will give you. It may take you a little longer and you may have to fit yourself into the role to achieve the same degree of responsiveness as the mother. All this can be helped by early and extended contact with your baby in her first weeks of life. Very often birth helps a man to express and enjoy emotions that society primes him to repress.

Establishing a routine

THE FIRST FEW DAYS will be hard; labour and birth are physically and emotionally draining. If you are in hospital you are subject to a certain amount of routine – regular checks by midwives, ward rounds by obstetricians or paediatricians, meals at certain times, visits by physiotherapists, family and friends, and so on – plus learning to feed, change and bath your baby. I had my first baby in hospital and expected to have a restful time; instead I hardly had a minute to myself, few minutes alone with my baby and was utterly exhausted at night – I couldn't wait to get home to peace and security.

Even if you have your baby at home, you'll find that one activity succeeds another almost without respite, and all the time you are learning. You may have read all the baby books that are available, but no book tells you about your baby. There's no short cut to learning about your baby's care because you have to take your lead

from her. Babies don't know night from day and they require the same attention during the night as they do during the day.

The smaller your baby, the more often you will have to feed her. Small babies, say 3.1kg (7lb) or under, require food at least every four hours and often there may be only three hours or two and a half hours between feeds. You should feed on demand; if you do, your baby will find her own routine faster than if you try to impose your routine on her. At least twice during the night your newborn baby will need a feed and a nappy change. Nearly everyone I have spoken to seems to have had a well-behaved baby who slept for six hours during the night within a week of being delivered. Well, mine didn't! The baby that gives you more than four hours' sleep during the night is an exception.

The best way to manage all that's demanded of you and to stay cheerful and to get enough rest is to take your cue from

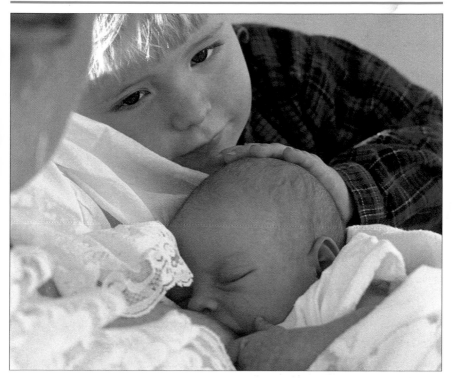

the baby. You're going to have to learn to catnap because the only opportunity you may get to sleep during the first few days is when your baby is asleep. Just after delivery you have little stamina and will easily become exhausted from physical effort. Emotionally you are in a labile state because of the sudden withdrawal of pregnancy hormones. Little problems seem insurmountable and big ones insoluble. You may find yourself short-tempered and irritable with flashes of elation in between. You may be tearful and collapse in a heap as soon as anything goes wrong and the next minute find yourself imbued with strong resolutions. Don't expect too much of yourself.

If you have a home confinement, or an early discharge from hospital, be easy on yourself. Don't worry about day-to-day domestic chores. Let them pile up; any

NEW MEMBER OF THE FAMILY
When you introduce your new baby to an older child, let him feel and touch her.

outside helper can see to those things. Save your energy to concentrate on what matters, and there really are only a few things that should get top priority: the baby, then you, then your partner and any other children, then all of you as a family unit. Be unscrupulous in asking for help, even if it's only for the first week, so that you have time on your own to get to know your baby and to work your day around her needs.

Most newborn babies have the same basic needs in the first few weeks of life, and once you have established a routine, you can then set about deciding what your needs are and how best to organize yourself on a typical day.

Rights and benefits

PREGNANT WOMEN are entitled to a range of rights and benefits depending on their circumstances and national insurance (NI) contributions. The entitlements, particularly for those on low incomes, are complicated but your Social Security office, Citizen's Advice Bureau or legal advice centre should be able to work out what you are eligible for.

If you are working, any maternity leave and pay from your employer must be explained to you by your employer or trade union representative. The chart below shows you how to get your maximum entitlement. If you need further information, contact your local Social Security office or Job Centre.

BENEFITS DURING PREGNANCY

Pregnant women are eligible for free NHS dental treatment and prescriptions, and you may get free milk and vitamins if you are on a low income. Statutory Maternity Pay (SMP) is operated by your employer and is not dependent on your going back to work. For mothers who can't get SMP because they are self-employed, have changed jobs or are not working, there is a maternity allowance payable for up to 26 weeks provided the qualifying conditions are satisfied.

If you are not entitled to SMP or Maternity Allowance, you may get eight weeks' incapacity benefit. Mothers who

WHEN	WHAT TO DO	WHY
AS SOON AS YOU KNOW YOU ARE PREGNANT	1 Ask your doctor for form FW8. 2 Tell your dentist. 3 Check leaflet HC 11 and tell your Social Security office if you are getting Income Support. 4 Tell your employer. 5 Find out about Maternity Allowance.	1 To apply for free prescriptions. 2 To get free dental treatment. 3 To check your right to free glasses, free milk and vitamins, and help with hospital fares. 4 To find out about SMP (Statutory Maternity Pay) and time off for antenatal appointments. 5 If you can't get SMP.
AS SOON AS YOU CAN	If you are unemployed or ill, ask your Social Security office about making a claim for Maternity Allowance.	It can affect the amount of Maternity Allowance you may get.
20 WEEKS OF PREGNANCY	1 Ask your doctor or midwife for a maternity certificate (form MAT B1) showing when your baby is due. 2 If you are employed, give MAT B1 to your employer. 3 If you cannot get SMP, ask at your maternity or child health clinic or Social Security office for form MA 1.	1 You need this form to qualify for SMP or Maternity Allowance. 2 To protect your right to SMP and allow your employer to work out your entitlement. If you delay later than 3 weeks after your SMP could have started, you may lose your SMP. 3 You can apply for Maternity Allowance on form MA 1.
15 WEEKS BEFORE THE EXPECTED DATE OF THE BIRTH	Tell your employer in writing when you will be stopping work; the week the baby is due; and whether you intend to return to your job.	To protect your right to SMP, maternity leave and the right to return to work at the end of the longer maternity absence.
29 WEEKS *Your 14 week maternity leave period can start now.*	Apply for a maternity payment from the Social Fund if you or your partner are on Income Support, Family Credit or Disability Working Allowance.	To pay for items for the baby.

are on Income Support or Family Credit, may get a maternity payment from the Social Fund. Women on their own after the baby is born get a tax-free weekly cash payment (on top of child benefit) regardless of income or NI contributions.

WORKING WOMEN

As a working woman, you are entitled by law to 26 weeks' maternity leave, however long you have worked for your employer. During this time you are entitled to all your normal terms of employment except wages or salary, and afterwards you can return to your job. The earliest you can start your leave is 11 weeks before the week that you expect your baby.

To qualify for SMP you must have been in the same employment for at least 26 weeks without a break by the 15th week before the week your baby is due, and you must have earned enough to pay Class 1 NI contributions. SMP is paid for up to 26 weeks. For the first 6 weeks you get 90% of your average weekly earnings and a flat rate after that. SMP may be liable to the deductions that are normally taken out of your wages.

In addition, additional maternity leave lasts for 26 weeks and starts at the end of ordinary maternity leave. You are entitled to additional maternity leave if you have worked for your employer for 26 weeks by the 15th week before your baby is due. It is important that you tell your employer what you are going to do, and make it clear if you wish to return to work so that your job is kept open for you. You are also entitled to paid time off to go to antenatal clinics and you are protected against unfair dismissal when pregnant.

WHEN	WHAT TO DO	WHY
AS SOON AFTER THE BIRTH AS POSSIBLE	1 Register the baby's birth. This must be done within 6 weeks (3 weeks in Scotland). 2 Send off form for Child Benefit and, if you are a single parent, for Lone Parent payment. 3 Ask about low income benefits.	1 To get the birth certificate and NHS card. 2 To get Child Benefit and Lone Parent payment. 3 To see if you qualify for extra income support; help with rent, council tax, dental treatment and hospital fares; and free prescriptions, milk and vitamins,
DURING YOUR MATERNITY LEAVE	1 Give your employer 7 days' notice if you want to go back to work before the end of your 14 weeks' maternity leave. If you want to go back to work at the end of 14 weeks' maternity leave, you do not need to do anything. 2 Reply in writing within 2 weeks to any letter from your employer asking if you are going back to work after the end of the longer maternity absence.	1 Your employer can postpone your return for up to 7 days if you do not tell him you want to go back early. 2 To protect your right to return to work by the end of the 28th week after the week your baby is born.
3 MONTHS AFTER THE BIRTH	If you or your partner are getting Income Support or Family Credit, apply for a maternity payment from Social Fund.	You will lose maternity payment from the Social Fund if not claimed by now.
3 WEEKS BEFORE RETURN TO WORK	Write to your employer stating that you wish to return.	To protect your right to return to work and to help your employer plan for your return.
29 WEEKS FROM THE BIRTH	Return to work as your maternity leave is officially over.	You may lose your right to return to work.
6 MONTHS AFTER THE BIRTH	Claim Child Benefit.	Latest date for claiming, if Child Benefit is to be paid from date of birth.

Useful addresses

The Active Birth Centre
25 Bickerton Road
London N19 5JT
☎ 020 7281 6760
www.activebirthcentre.com
Information and classes for those who seek to avoid a high-tech birth.

AcuMedic
101–105 Camden High Street
London NW1 7JN
☎ 020 7388 6704
www.acumedic.com
Advice on acupuncture and fertility.

Action on Pre-eclampsia
84-88 Pinner Road
Harrow HA1 4HZ
☎ 020 8863 3271
www.apec.org.uk
Advice on pre-eclampsia.

Association of Breastfeeding Mothers
PO Box 207
Bridgwater TA6 7YT
☎ 0870 401 7711
www.abm.me.uk
24-hour counselling service.

Association for Improvements in Maternity Services (AIMS)
5 Anne's Court
Grove Road
Surbiton KT6 4BE
☎ 0870 765 1453
0870 765 1433 (helpline)
www.aims.org.uk
Provides support and information about maternity choices.

Association for Spina Bifida and Hydrocephalus (ASBAH)
Asbah House, 42 Park Road
Peterborough
PE1 2UQ
☎ 01733 555988
www.asbah.org
Information and advice for parents of children with spina bifida.

**BLISS
(Baby Life Support Systems)**
68 South Lambeth Road
London SW8 1RL
☎ 020 7820 9471
0500 618 140 (helpline)
www.bliss.org.uk
Helpline for parents of special care babies.

British Acupuncture Council
63 Jeddo Road
London W12 9HQ
☎ 020 8735 0400
www.acupuncture.org.uk
Provides a list of qualified practitioners.

British Homeopathic Association
Hahnemann House
29 Park Street West
Luton LU1 3BE
☎ 0870 444 3950
www.trusthomeopathy.org

British Liver Trust
Portman House
44 High Street
Ringwood BH24 1AG
☎ 01425 463080
www.britishlivertrust.org.uk
Information and advice on liver disease in pregnancy.

The Compassionate Friends
53 North Street
Bristol BS3 1EN
☎ 0117 966 5202
0845 232304 (helpline)
www.tcf.org.uk
Puts bereaved parents in touch with others who have had a similar experience.

Contact a Family
209-211 City Road
London EC1V 1JN
☎ 020 7608 8700
0808 808 3555 (helpline)
www.cafamily.org.uk
Puts parents of children with special needs in touch with others.

CRY-SIS Support Group
BM Cry-Sis
London WC1N 3XX
☎ 020 7404 5011
www.cry-sis.org.uk
Advice on babies who cry excessively.

Down's Syndrome Association
Langdon Down Centre
2a Langdon Park
Teddington TW11 9PS
☎ 0845 230 0372
www.downs-syndrome.org.uk
Advice on the care and treatment of people with Down's syndrome.

fpa (The Family Planning Association)
2–12 Pentonville Road
London N1 9FP
☎ 020 7837 5432
0845 310 1334 (helpline)
www.fpa.org.uk

The Foundation for the Study of Infant Deaths
11-19 Artillery Row
London SW1P 1RT
☎ 0870 787 0885
0870 787 0554 (helpline)
www.sids.org.uk/fsid
Researches the causes of cot death and provides support for parents.

Gingerbread
7 Sovereign Close
London E1W 2HW
☎ 020 7488 9300
0800 018 4318 (helpline)
www.gingerbread.org.uk
Support for one-parent families.

Independent Midwives' Association
1 The Great Quarry
Guildford GU1 3XN
☎ 01483 821104
www.independentmidwives.org.uk
Network of independent midwives offering private care.

La Leche League (Great Britain)
PO Box 29
West Bridgford
Nottingham NG2 7NP
☎ 0845 120 2918 (helpline)
www.laleche.org.uk
*Help and information for mothers
who want to breastfeed.*

The Lady
39–40 Bedford Street
London WC2E 9ER
☎ 020 7379 4717
www.lady.co.uk
*Magazine with advertisements for
nannies, mother's helps and au pairs.*

**Marie Stopes House Family
Planning Clinic**
153–157 Cleveland Street
London WIT 6QW
☎ 020 7574 7400
www.mariestopes.org.uk
*Information and advice about
family planning, sterilization etc.*

The Maternity Alliance
Third Floor West
2–6 Northburgh Street
London EC1V 0AY
☎ 020 7490 7639
020 7490 7638 (information)
www.maternityalliance.org.uk
*Information on all aspects of
maternity rights and benefits.*

MENCAP
123 Golden Lane
London EC1Y 0RT
☎ 020 7454 0454
www.mencap.org.uk
*Support for families of children and
adults with learning difficulties.*

The Miscarriage Association
c/o Clayton Hospital
Northgate, Wakefield
West Yorkshire WF1 3JS
☎ 01924 200799 (helpline)
www.miscarriageassociation.org.uk
*Help, advice and support for those
who have had a miscarriage.*

National Childbirth Trust
Alexandra House
Oldham Terrace
London W3 6NH
☎ 0870 4448707
www.nctpregnancyandbabycare.com
*Organizes antenatal classes
nationwide and offers help after the
baby is born.*

**National Childminding
Association**
8 Masons Hill
Bromley, Kent BR2 9EY
☎ 020 8464 6164
www.ncma.org.uk
*Organization of those with an interest
in pre-school care of babies and
children to improve the status of
minders and facilities for the children.*

One Parent Families
255 Kentish Town Road
London NW5 2LX
☎ 020 7428 5400
0800 018 5026 (helpline)
www.oneparentfamilies.org.uk
Advice for one-parent families.

**The National Meet-a-Mum
Association (MAMA)**
376 Bideford Green, Linslade,
Leighton Buzzard, LU7 2TY
☎ 01525 217064
*Help for new mothers, particularly
those suffering postnatal depression.*

**Royal College of
Obstetricians & Gynaecologists**
27 Sussex Place
London NW1 4RG
☎ 020 7772 6200
www.rcog.org.uk

Parentline Plus
520 Highgate Studios
53–79 Highgate Road
London NW5 1TL
020 7284 5536
☎ 0808 800 2222 (helpline)
www.parentlineplus.org.uk
Support for parents and carers.

Royal College of Midwives
15 Mansfield Street
London W1G 9NH
☎ 020 7312 3535
www.rcm.org.uk

**Stillbirth and Neonatal
Death Society (SANDS)**
28 Portland Place
London W1B 1LY
☎ 020 7436 7940
020 7436 5881 (helpline)
www.uk-sands.org

Scope
PO Box 833
Milton Keynes MK12 5NY
☎ 0800 800 3333 (helpline)
www.scope.org.uk
*Information and support for people
with cerebral palsy and their families.*

**St Mary's Hospital Recurrent
Miscarriage Clinic**
Winston Churchill Wing
Praed Street
London W2 1NY
☎ 020 7886 6000

**Twins and Multiple Births
Association (TAMBA)**
2 The Willows
Gardner Road
Guildford, Surrey
GU1 4PG
☎ 0870 770 3305
www.tamba.org.uk
*A self-help organization offering
encouragement and support before
and after multiple births.*

Wellbeing
27 Sussex Place
London NW1 4SP
☎ 020 7772 6400
www.wellbeing.demon.co.uk
*Funds research for better health for
women and babies and development
of new treatments for problems
during and after birth.*

Index

Index

G

Gas and air analgesia 135, 138
General practitioner (GP) units 27
Genetic diseases, amniocentesis check 52, 53
German measles (rubella) 45
Gums 63

H

Haemoglobin 45, 60
Haeomophilia 51, 53
Hair 63, 98
Head exercise 89
Health and fitness
  after childbirth 24
  exercises for 80ñ93
  in pregnancy 44-5, 70-7, 80, 82
Heart
  fetal and newborn 44
  maternal 61
Height of mother 44
High blood pressure
  (hypertension), in pregnancy 45
Hip exercise 89
HIV tests 45
Home, preparing for baby 108-9
Home delivery 27, 28-9, 46, 112-13, 115
Hormones
  effects on hair 63
  effects on skin 62, 98
  follicle-stimulating hormone (FSH) 54
  human chorionic gonadotrophin (HCG) 19, 20, 49, 55, 56
  human placental lactogen (HPL) 56
  melanocyte stimulating hormone (MSH) 56
  mood changes and 64
  oestrogen 19, 55
  ovarian 54, 56
  pituitary 54
  placental 55
  in pregnancy 18-19, 54-6
  progesterone 19, 55, 84
  relaxin 56
Hospitals
  admission procedure 118
  antenatal clinics 42, 43, 46
  birth 27, 30-3, 35-8, 113, 115
  delivery room 38
  maternity units 27
  what to take 113
Human chorionic gonadotrophin (HCG) 19, 20, 55, 56

Hypertension see High blood pressure
Hypnosis, pain relief 137

I

Immunization, rubella 45
Implantation of embryo 54
Incontinence, urinary 84
Induction of labour 140-1
Infections, sex and 68, 69
Inhalation analgesia 135, 138
Insomnia 100
Intelligence and parental bonding 150
Internal examination, in labour 121
Iron 60, 75-6, 77
  supplements 45, 46, 76
Itching 98

J

Joints 61, 80

K

Kegel (pelvic floor) exercises 84-5
Kidneys 61
  infections 44
Kitzinger, Sheila, episiotomy survey 139

L

Labour see Childbirth and labour
Lactation see Breasts; Breastfeeding
Lamaze, Fernand 33
Leboyer, Frederick 33-4
Leg exercises 87
Lifting 81
Ligaments 61, 80
Linea nigra 62
Looks 94-9
Lungs 61
Lying positions 106

M

Make-up 98, 99
Malformations see Abnormal babies
Massage 105
Maternal bonding 39, 148-50
Melanocyte stimulating hormone (MSH) 56

Membrane rupture 117, 140-1
Menstrual cycle 54-5, 56
Menstruation
  after childbirth 24
  delivery date (EDD) and 42
  missed period (amenorrhoea) 19
  suppression in pregnancy 55
Metabolic disease, amniocentesis and 53
Metabolism 100
Midwives 27, 29, 32, 47, 121
Milk see Breast milk; Cow's milk
Minerals 61, 75-7
  see also Iron
Miscarriage 55
  amniocentesis and 53
  intercourse and 69
  smoking and 78
Monitoring, electronic fetal (EFM) 118, 121, 142-3
Montgomery's tubercles 57
Monthly cycle 55, 56
Mood changes 64
Morning sickness 19, 56
Multiple pregnancy
  ultrasound detection 51
  see also Twins
Muscular dystrophy 53

N

Nails 63
Nappies 110
Narcotics 138
National Childbirth Trust (NCT) 33
Natural childbirth movement 33-5
Nausea 19, 56
Neck exercise 89
Neural tube defects 49
Nipples 56
  changes in pregnancy 19, 57, 62
  inverted or flat 44, 57
Nuchal translucency scan 51
Nursery and equipment 108-11
Nutrition of mother
  foods to avoid 73
  in pregnancy 44, 61, 63, 70-7
  vital nutrients 74-7
  vulnerable women 75
  weight gain 72

O

Obesity 72
Obstetricians 27, 32-3, 43, 47
Odent, Michel 34-5
Oedema 44, 74

Acknowledgments

2005 edition
Dorling Kindersley would like to thank Sarah Reynolds MD MRCOG for her advice on current practices in pregnancy, childbirth and baby care, Connie Novis for proofreading, and the following people for modelling for photographs: Mark Adams and Clare Massie, Cathy Barratt with Alexandra, Anna Dawson with Ben, Lalaine Edson, Liz Mischka with Felix, the Moody family, Nora Musitwa, Birgul Mustafa, Sarah-Jane and Andrew Wood, Patrick, Mars, Poppy and Tom. Dorling Kindersley would also like to thank Vicki Barnes and Louise Heywood for help with hair and make-up.

ILLUSTRATION

Edwina Keene, Jenny Powell, David Lawrence, Kuo Kang Chen, Coral Mula, Trevor Hill

PHOTOGRAPHY

Dorling Kindersley would like to thank Ruth Jenkinson for the photographs on pages 66, 71, 81, 91, 95, 96, 97, 99, 101, 104-105, 106-107, 114, 123, 125, 126.

They are also grateful to the following for permission to reproduce their photographs: Andy Crawford: 83; Anthea Sieveking/Wellcome Photo Library: 1, 2, 28, 31, 37, 132, 133; Chris Harvey 102; Corbis/Cameron: 215; Masterfile/B Kuhlmann: 2; Mother & Baby Picture Library/emap élan: 9, 10, 11, 12, 13, 14, 15, 16, 17; Mother & Baby Picture Library/Ian Hooten: 46, 47 (left), 47 (right); Mother & Baby Picture Library/P Mitchell: 109; Mother & Baby Picture Library/Ruth Jenkinson: 121, 122, 135; Nancy Durrell McKenna: 128-129, 130; Phillip & Karen Smith 151; Ronald Mckechnie (right); Roger Tully 43; Science Photo Library/BSIP/ Laurent/Laura: 50; Science Photo Library/BSIP/Astier: 52; Science Photo Library/Ruth Jenkinson: 142; Telegraph Colour Library: Antonio Mo 65; Tony Stone Images: Bruce Ayres 118.